Anthology of Orthopaedics

Anthology
of Orthopaedics

MERCER RANG FRCS

Orthopaedic Surgeon
The Hospital for Sick Children
Toronto, Canada

CHURCHILL LIVINGSTONE
EDINBURGH LONDON AND NEW YORK 1966

CHURCHILL LIVINGSTONE
Medical Division of Longman Group Limited

Distributed in the United States of America by
Churchill Livingstone Inc., 19 West 44th Street, New York,
N.Y. 10036 and by associated companies, branches and
representatives throughout the world.

First Edition 1966
Reprinted 1968
Reprinted 1977
Reprinted 1980
ISBN 0 443 00408 0

**Library of Congress Cataloging in Publication
Data**
The Library of Congress Cataloged the First Issue of
This Title as Follows:

Rang, Mercer, *ed.*
   Anthology of orthopaedics. Edinburgh, E. & S.
Livingstone, 1966.

   xi, 242 p. illus., plates, ports. 26 cm.
   Bibliography: p. 233–237.

   1. Orthopedia—Address, essays, lectures.   1. Title.
[RD721]   617.3008   66–1508/CD

Printed in Hong Kong by
Wah Cheong Printing Press Ltd.

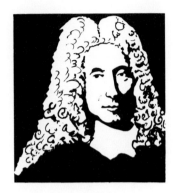

ORTHOPAEDIA

As to the Title, I have formed it of two Greek words, viz. ORTHOS, which signifies straight, free from deformity, and PAIS, a child.

Out of these two words, I have compounded that of ORTHOPAEDIA, to express in one term the design I propose, which is to teach the different methods of preventing and correcting deformities of children.

Nicholas Andry, 1741

PREFACE

"There's a Pott's fracture for you!"

"I don't know what you mean by 'a Pott's fracture'," said Alice.

"I meant, there's 'a nice fractured ankle' for you!"

"But, a Pott's fracture doesn't mean 'a nice fractured ankle'," Alice objected.

"When I use a word," Humpty Dumpty said in a rather scornful tone, "It means just what I choose it to mean—neither more nor less." (With apologies to Lewis Carroll.)

Once a name becomes a cliché, everyone is free to interpret it as they wish. So many diseases, physical signs and methods of treatment known after famous men, particularly in orthopaedics, have become clichés. Their original meaning is lost in the past or lies between the unopened covers of an almost forgotten book. I am not greatly in favour of eponymous names, but, if they are to be retained, they should be used with accuracy. If medical textbooks are to serve as Rolls of Honour, the gravestones should carry the correct names. Opponents to this form of ancestor worship must not be allowed to destroy it by making it vague and meaningless, but should be encouraged to use the alternative descriptive title.

How can meaning and definition be restored? Not by asking, and not by reading current works, but only by studying the original. This is not easy: the original is often hard to find (as there are only a few cities in the world with suitable libraries) and may be written in another language. Because of the difficulties, few people have the time or opportunity to read for themselves the articles that have added new words to the language or new ideas to surgical thinking.

The intention of this book is to give new life to classical orthopaedic literature—to make it available once more. This is a guide book; the contents have been selected for their interest without attempting to be comprehensive. Most of the papers have been reproduced only in part, in order to compile a book of manageable size. Many subjects have not been touched upon: some were too long; some did not catch my attention, and some subjects have seen such a slow build-up of knowledge that no particular account is outstanding.

Rather than produce an encyclopaedia, I have tried to produce an un-believably good volume of an orthopaedic journal. One of the subconscious pleasures of reading a current journal is that it enables the reader to discover the activities of his friends and rivals. This link is missing when one goes into the past. In order to recreate this, I have included biographies and portraits of the authors. Most of them were men of the greatest eminence. I say this once, at the beginning, because in trying to bring them alive again I dealt with them anecdotally, and perhaps irreverently, since a catalogue of their honours and distinctions reduces their individual calibre, and may make one distinguished man very like another. Serious students of biography will find a list of references to more formal material at the end.

The idea for this anthology came whilst I was working for Lipmann Kessel, Esq., whose stimulating teaching is often enlivened by historical reference. Without the atmosphere he generated, and the encouragement he gave, this would never have been completed. Much of the anthology was written at the Royal National Orthopaedic Hospital where the facilities available were of great help to me. I wish to thank Robert Whitley, F.R.P.S. for preparing the illustrations and my portrait sketches for publication, C. Davenport, B.Sc., A.R.C.S., the Librarian, for helping me find much of the material; the Librarians at University College Hospital Medical School, The Wellcome Historical Medical Library, The Royal College of Surgeons of England and the Université de Paris were all very helpful. Translations were prepared by my neighbours Dieter Pevsner and Dr. H. J. Hirsch, Dr. J. Wicht and my wife. Miss Morrant Baker kindly lent me a portrait of her father. Colonel Metz, U.S.M.S. sent me a memoir and portrait of Keller. My mother and my wife prepared the typescript. Dr. Derek Kirkpatrick read some of the proofs. I am grateful to the following for permission to reproduce copyright material:

Baillière, Tindall & Cox, Ltd.: Jules Tinel, *Nerve Wounds.*

Capelli: M. Ortolani, *La Lussazione congenita dell anca.*

Longmans Green & Co. Ltd.: R. A. Stafford, *The Injuries, the Diseases, Distortions of the Spine.*

Oxford University Press: T. P. McMurray, *Robert Jones Birthday Volume.*

Archiv für orthopädische und Unfall-Chirurgie; Berliner klinische Wochenschrift; British Journal of Surgery; Bulletin et mémoires de la Société de médicale Hôpiteaux de Paris; Deutsche medizinische Wochenschrift; Glasgow Medical Journal; Journal of Bone and Joint Surgery; Korrespondenzblatt für schweizer Arzte; The Lancet; New England Journal of Medicine; Presse médicale; Proceedings of the Royal Society; Revue de médecine; St. Bartholomew's Hospital Reports; Surgery, Gynecology & Obstetrics; Verhandlungen der deutschen gesellschaft für Chirurgie; Verhandlungen naturhistorich-medizinische Vereins; Zeitschrift orthopädische Chirurgie.

Finally, Mr. Charles Macmillan and Livingstones deserve my gratitude for turning a manuscript into a finely produced book.

To all these kindly, generous and helpful people I offer my sincere thanks.

Kingston, Jamaica, 1965.   M.R.

CONTENTS

Note: Names in capitals indicate a biography and portrait.

Part Three

PATHOLOGY

Part Four

PHYSICAL SIGNS

As some delight most to behold;
  Each new device and guise,
So some in works of fathers old,
  Their studies exercise.

Perusing with all diligence,
  Books written long before,
Wherein they learn experience,
  To heal both sick and sore.

Which I allow in deed and word,
  In those that understand:
For otherwise it is a sword,
  Put in a mad man's hand..

Lanfranke's CHIRURGICAL WORKES 1565

PART ONE
GENERAL LANDMARKS

GENERAL LANDMARKS

Orthopaedics, as part of medicine, depends to a great extent on basic discoveries, such as the understanding of anatomy and physiology, antisepsis, anaesthesia and so on. The juxtaposition of these advances and of new ideas in orthopaedics gives the history of orthopaedic surgery many odd twists and turns.

Operations on bones and joints have been carried out for centuries, reaching a high degree of sophistication by the early nineteenth century. Osteotomy, arthroplasty and major amputations featured in the repertoire of surgeons of this period, though anaesthesia, antiseptics and blood transfusion had not been introduced. The mortality from these procedures transformed them into a surgical lottery; however, the germ of an idea was waiting until the situation was more suitable for it to flower. Surgical ideas were ahead of the techniques essential for their success. For example, Langenbeck nailed a hip fracture in 1850 but the metal corroded. A fractured humerus was wired together in 1775 but infection killed the patient.

What are these techniques to which the modern patient, expecting a reliable outcome from his treatment, owes so much? They repay a little attention as their chronology does much to explain the evolution of practical orthopaedics.

1. *Anaesthesia*

Anaesthesia was introduced in the eighteen-forties in America. The early history and claims for priority are a little confused and acrimonious but it was certainly William T. G. Morton, a Boston dentist, who realised its tremendous worth at the end of 1846. Within a couple of months it was used in London, and quickly anaesthesia based on nitrous oxide, ether, and chloroform, was being widely administered.

2. *Aseptic Surgery*

In 1865 Lord Lister performed his first operation using *anti*septic surgery and two years later he described the technique before the annual meeting of the British Medical Association.

"Previously to its introduction the two large wards in which most of my cases of accident and operation are treated were among the unhealthiest in the whole surgical division of the Glasgow Royal Infirmary, in consequence apparently of those wards being unfavourably placed with reference to the supply of fresh air: and I have felt ashamed when recording the results of my practice, to have so often to allude to hospital gangrene or pyaemia. It was interesting, though melancholy, to observe that whenever all or nearly all the beds contained cases with open sores, these grievous complications were pretty sure to show themselves; so that I came to welcome simple fractures, though in themselves of little interest either for myself or the students, because their presence diminished the proportion of open sores among the patients. But since the antiseptic treatment has been brought into full operation, and wounds and abscesses no longer poison the atmosphere with putrid exhalations, my wards, though in other respects under precisely the same circumstances as before, have completely changed their character; so that during the last nine months not a single case of pyaemia, hospital gangrene, or erysipelas has occurred in them."

Despite Lister's claim antiseptic surgery took many years to establish itself. The younger surgeons accepted his ideas but the older ones often carried on as they always had.

3. *Radiology*

Just before Christmas 1895, Wilhelm Röntgen (1845-1923), Professor of Physics at Würzburg, found that when he passed a high voltage current through a Crookes vacuum tube, a ray was generated which would pass through cardboard, wood and limbs. He demonstrated this at a meeting at Würzburg and proposed that the rays should be called 'X-Ray'. The president of the meeting suggested Röntgen rays.

Within weeks of the discovery of X-rays they came into medical use. For example, Robert Jones was sent a press cutting about them by a patient. He went straight to Würzburg and came back with a set which he installed in 11, Nelson Street. At first X-rays were used for discovering metallic foreign bodies but as the equipment improved over the next 10 years X-rays came into wider use.

4. *Metallurgy*

It was only about 30 years ago that electrolytic corrosion was realised to be a major problem affecting metallic implants. The original trouble with metal implants was the same as it is today, namely, the risk of infection entailed by inserting a foreign body at open operation. It is salutary to note that even in 1775 surgeons were arguing about internal fixation, along the same lines, but with more point, as they do today.

For orthopaedic use a metal must be strong, workable, and free from tissue reaction. The precious metals were popular in the nineteenth century but were rather soft. Lane in 1894 used steel and stated that he never saw a tissue reaction. Steel does not corrode in the tissues as badly as other metals and he did not mix metals which produces the most rapid disintegration. However, other people using Lane's equipment found that they frequently had to remove the metal. This gave rise to the still widely held belief that all metals should be removed after serving their purpose. Once Lane had demonstrated that internal fixation of fractures was both sound and safe, a large number of surgeons developed the idea, many of them using two different metals for the operation. Reactions were common. In

3

1925 a surgeon was applying an aluminium plate to a fracture of the humerus near the radial nerve; every time he touched the plate with his brass screws, the fingers extended.

The use of materials was empirical until Charles Venable and Walter Stuck began studying the problem of corrosion in the nineteen-thirties. One of the better materials was stainless steel. This was first invented by Harry Breasley in 1913. Later in 1926 one of the many variants, 18-8 S. Mo. Stainless Steel was introduced. It consisted of 18 per cent. chromium, 8-10 per cent. nickel and 2-4 per cent. molybdenum. Venable and Stuck found that this material, which was fairly popular, was better than most, but still corroded to a very limited extent.

A dental friend introduced them to vitallium while they were carrying out this study, because it did not corrode in the mouth. Vitallium, a non-ferrous alloy composed of 65 per cent. cobalt, 30 per cent. chromium, and 3 per cent. molybdenum, had been developed in 1929. On chemical and animal tests they found it more inert than stainless steel and started to use it clinically in 1936.

Since then stainless steel and vitallium have become the standard. Corrosion is hardly a problem.

5. *Antibiotics*

Sulphonamides paved the way in 1935 but were unfortunately not very active against the organisms of orthopaedic significance. Penicillin was a war time development. The antituberculous and wide spectrum drugs were introduced after the war.

The reduction of chronic infection is to a large degree due to the antibiotics, though better nutrition, and conditions of living have helped.

6. *Vaccines*

Vaccines have changed the face of orthopaedics. In the First World War tetanus vaccine came into use and drastically cut this complication of trauma. In the fifties Salk and then Sabin polio vaccine were used and have almost eradicated this problem.

It is now time to turn to the original papers. Just as many of the basic techniques were worked out by people other than orthopaedic surgeons, so we will find that many of the diseases and physical signs were described by physicians, neurologists, chiropodists, general practitioners, radiologists, and general surgeons.

PART TWO

CLASSIC DESCRIPTIONS OF DISEASE

1 INFECTIONS

Spinal Tuberculosis: Hippocrates

Hippocrates is an almost faceless, unknown man who has left a wonderful collection of works known after him. The collection, written in the 3rd and 4th centuries B.C., is at once the first medical book of note and the most important work for the next two millenia. Most of today's aids to treatment have come in over the last 100 years: for example, anaesthesia, X-rays, asepsis, antibiotics, blood transfusion; this development has occurred over a period that is about one-twentieth of that during which Hippocrates' works remained standard teaching. Yet his works were not printed until the Renaissance and were not translated into English until the last century.

The legend is that he was born in Cos, an island in the eastern Aegean off the Turkish coast, about 460 B.C., and later travelled widely, though living mainly in Cos, where, under a plane tree, he taught his students until his death about 355 B.C. Portraits of him probably depict someone else.

Hippocrates was a very critical observer of disease, and wrote one book on fractures and another on articulations which repay reading. They are systematic works containing so much of value that it is difficult to itemise.

Hippocrates: 3rd Century B.C.

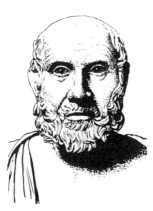

The vertebrae of the spine, when contracted into a lump behind from disease, for the most part cannot be remedied; more especially when the gibbosity is above the attachment of the diaphragm to the spine.

When the gibbosity occurs in youth before the body is fully grown, spinal growth stops, but the arms and legs are fully developed. And in those cases where the gibbosity is above the diaphragm, the ribs do not usually expand properly in width, but forwards, and the chest becomes short, pointed and not broad. They become affected by difficulty of breathing and hoarseness as the cavities which inspire and expire the breath do not attain their proper capacity. They generally have hard and unconcocted tubercles in the lungs, for the gibbosity and swelling in the neck are mostly produced by such tubercles. When the gibbosity is below the diaphragm in some of these cases, nephritic diseases and affections of the bladder supervene, chronic abscesses that are difficult to cure occur in the loins and groins, and neither of these removes the gibbosity. In these cases

6

the hips are more emaciated than when the gibbosity is seated higher up; the hair of the pubes and chin is of slower growth and less developed, and they are less capable of generation than those with the gibbosity higher up.

Percivall Pott, 1714-1788

Percivall Pott's father came from a London family who were so prolific that it was a standing joke among their friends that although they were green-grocers by trade, they were the best Pott makers in London.

Percivall Pott was a Cockney born in Threadneedle Street, London, and was apprenticed to a surgeon at St. Bartholomew's Hospital. He obtained the Grand Diploma of the Barber Surgeon's Company in 1736, and was appointed to the staff of St. Bartholomew's eight years later. He soon established himself as a teacher and a humane surgeon. His son-in-law gives this account of the famous injury which lead him to start writing:

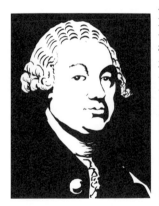

In the year 1756, an accident befell Mr. Pott. As he was riding in Kent Street, Southwark, he was thrown from his horse, and suffered a compound fracture of the leg, the bone being forced through the integuments. Conscious of the dangers attendant on fractures of this nature, and thoroughly aware how much they may be increased by rough treatment, or improper position, he would not suffer himself to be moved until he had made the necessary dispositions. He sent to Westminster, then the nearest place, for two chairmen, to bring their poles; and patiently lay on the cold pavement, it being the middle of January, till they arrived. In this situation he purchased a door, to which he made them nail their poles. When all was ready, he caused himself to be laid on it, and was carried through South-wark, over London bridge, to Watling-street near St. Paul's, where he had lived for some time—a tremendous distance in such a state! I cannot forbear remarking, that on such occasions a coach is too frequently employed, the jolting motion of which, with the unavoid-able awkwardness of position and the difficulty of getting in and out, cause a great, and often a fatal aggravation of the mischief. At a consultation of surgeons, the case was thought so desperate as to require immediate amputation. Mr. Pott, convinced that no one could be a proper judge in his own case, submitted to their opinion; and the instruments were actually got ready, when Mr. Nourse, who had been prevented from coming sooner, fortunately entered the room. After examining the limb, he conceived there was a possibility of preserving it: an attempt to save it was acquiesced in, and succeeded. This case, which Mr. Pott sometimes referred to, was a strong instance of the great advantage of preventing the insinuation of air into the wound of a compound fracture; and it probably would not have ended so happily, if the bone had not made its exit, or external opening, at a distance from the fracture; so that, when it was returned into the proper place, a sort of valve was formed, which excluded air. Thus no bad symptom ensued, but the wound healed, in some measure, by the first intention.— The appearance of Mr. Pott as an author was an immediate effect of this accident. During the leisure of his necessary confinement, he planned, and partly executed his treatise upon ruptures, which was completed by the latter end of the year.

The site of the fracture is not mentioned, but as the fracture was at a distance from the skin wound it is more likely to have been a fracture of the shaft of the tibia than a Pott's fracture.

He wrote a classic monograph on head injuries and another on fractures and dislocations, drawing attention to the importance of relaxing the muscles which maintained deformity by correct positioning.

His account of tuberculous paraplegia was first published in 1779. He recognised the tuberculous nature of the disease but thought the paraplegia was due, not to cord compression, but to a distemper of the area. He advised drainage to stop the disease progressing and allow bony healing to take place.

He was a discursive writer, and this account is a curtailed version.

Pott's Paraplegia: 1779

REMARKS
ON THAT KIND OF
PALSY OF THE LOWER LIMBS,
which is frequently found to accompany
A CURVATURE OF THE SPINE
and is
supposed to be caused by it,
together
WITH ITS METHOD OF CURE

The disease of which I am to speak is a disease of the spine, producing an alteration in its natural figure, and not infrequently attended with a partial, or a total loss of the power of using, or even moving, the lower limbs.

From this last circumstance (the loss of the use of the limbs), it has in general been called a palsy, and treated as a paralytic affection; to which it is in almost every respect perfectly unlike.

The occasion of the mistake is palpable; the patient is deprived of the use of his legs, and has a deformed incurvation of the spine; the incurvation is supposed to be caused by a dislocation of the vertebrae; the displaced bones are thought to make an unnatural pressure on the spinal marrow; and a pressure on that being very likely to produce a paralysis of some kind, the loss of the use of the legs is in this case determined to be such. The truth is, that there is no dislocation, no unnatural pressure made on the spinal marrow; nor are the limbs by any means paralytic, as will appear to whoever will examine the two complaints with any degree of attention.

In the true paralysis, from whatever cause, the muscles of the affected limb are soft, flabby, unresisting, and incapable of being put into even a tonic state.

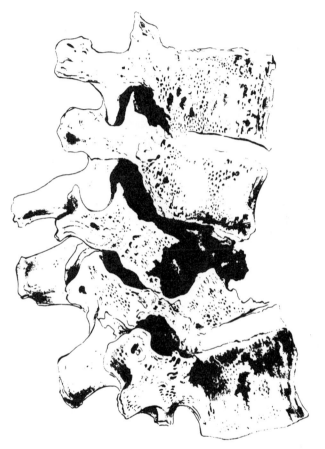

Pott's Disease

In the present case, the muscles are indeed extenuated, and lessened in size; but they are rigid, and always at least in a tonic state, by which the knees and ancles acquire a stiffness not very easy to overcome. By means of this stiffness, mixed with a kind of spasm, the legs of the patient are either constantly kept stretched out straight, in which case considerable force is required to bend the knees, or they are by the action of the stronger muscles drawn across each other in such manner as to require as much to separate them: when the leg is in a straight position, the extensor muscles act so powerfully as to require a considerable degree of force to bend the joints of the knees; and when they have been bent, the legs are immediately and strongly drawn up, with the heels towards the buttocks: by the rigidity of the ancle-joints, joined to the spasmodic action of the gastrocnemii muscles, the patient's toes are pointed downward in such manner as to render it impossible for him to put his foot flat to the ground; which makes one of the decisive characteristics of the distemper.

The majority of those who labour under this disease are infants or young children: adults are by no means exempt from it; but I have never seen it at an age beyond forty.

If the incurvation be of the neck, and to a considerable degree, by affecting several vertebrae, the child finds it inconvenient and painful to support its own head, and is always desirous of laying it on a table or pillow, or any thing to take off the weight. If the affection be of the dorsal vertebrae, the general marks of a distempered habit, such as loss of appetite, hard dry cough, laborious respiration, quick pulse, and disposition to hectic, appear pretty early, and in such a manner as to demand attention; and as in this state of the case there is always, from the connexion between the ribs, sternum, and spine, a great degree of crookedness of the trunk, these complaints are by every body set to the account of the deformity merely. In an adult, the attack and the progress of the disease are much the same, but there are some few circumstances which may be learned from a patient of such age, which either do not make an impression on a child, or do not happen to it.

An adult, in a case where no violence hath been committed, or received, will tell you, that his first intimation was a sense of weakness in his back-bone, accompanied with what he will call a heavy dull kind of pain, attended with such a lassitude as rendered a small degree of exercise fatiguing; that this was soon followed by an unusual sense of coldness in the thighs, not accountable for from the weather, and a palpable diminution of their sensibility; that, in a little time more, his limbs were frequently convulsed by involuntary twitchings, particularly troublesome in the night; that soon after this, he not only became incapable of walking, but that his power either of retaining or discharging his urine and faeces was considerably impaired, and his penis incapable of erection.

The primary and sole cause of all the mischief, is a distempered state of the parts composing or in immediate connection with the spine, tending to, and most frequently ending in, a caries of the body, or bodies, of one or more of the vertebrae: from this proceed all the ills, whether general or local, apparent or concealed; this causes the ill health of the patient, and, in time, the curvature. The helpless state of the limbs is only one consequence of several proceeding from the same cause: but though this effect is a very frequent one, and always affects the limbs in nearly the same manner, yet the disease not having its origin in them, no application made to them only can ever be of any possible use.

The same failure of success attends the use of the different pieces of machinery, and for reasons which are equally obvious.

They are founded upon the supposition of an actual *dislocation*, which never is the case, and therefore they always have been, and ever must be, unsuccessful.

To understand this in the clearest and most convincing manner, we need only reflect on the nature of the disease, its seat, and the state in which the parts concerned must necessarily be.

The bones are already carious, or tending to become so; the parts connected with them are diseased, and not infrequently ulcerated; there is no displacement of the vertebrae with regard to each other; and the spine bends forward only because the rotten bone, or bones intervening between the sound ones, give way, being unable in such state to bear the weight of the parts above.

These different affections of the spine, and of the parts in its immediate neighbourhood, are productive of many disorders, general and local, affecting the whole frame and habit of the patient, as well as particular parts; and, among the rest, of that curvature which is the subject of this inquiry; and it may not be amiss to remark, that strumous tubercles in the lungs, and a distempered state of some of the abdominal viscera, often make a part of them.

From an attentive examination of these morbid appearances, and of their effects in different subjects, and under different circumstances, the following observations, tending not only to illustrate and explain the true nature of the disease in question, but also to throw light on others of equal importance, may, I think, be made.

1. That the disease which produces these effects on the spine, and the parts in its vicinity, is what is in general called the scrophula; that is, the same kind of indisposition as occasions the thick upper lip, the tedious obstinate ophthalmy, the indurated glands under the chin and in the neck, the obstructed mesentery, the hard dry cough, the glairy swellings of the wrist and ancles, the thickened ligaments of the joints, the enlargement and caries of the bones, etc., etc., etc.

2. That this disease, by falling on the spine, and the parts connected with it, is the cause of a great variety of complaints, both general and local.

3. That when these complaints are not attended with an alteration of the figure of the backbone, neither the real seat, nor true nature of such distemper are pointed out by the general symptoms; and consequently, that they frequently are unknown, at least while the patient lives.

4. That when by means of this distemper an alteration is produced in the figure of the backbone, that alteration is different in different subjects, and according to different circumstances.

5. That when the ligaments and cartilages of the spine become the seat of the disorder, without any affection of the vertebrae, it sometimes happens that the whole spine, from the lowest vertebrae of the neck downwards, gives way laterally, forming sometimes one great curve to one side, and sometimes a more irregular figure, producing general crookedness and deformity of the whole trunk of the body, attended with many marks of ill health.

6. That these complaints, which are by almost every body

supposed to be the effect of the deformity merely, are really occasioned by that distempered state of the parts within the thorax, which is at the same time the cause both of the deformity and of the want of health.

7. That the attack is sometimes on the bodies of some of the vertebrae; and that when this is the case, ulceration or erosion of the bone is the consequence, and not enlargement.

8. That when this erosion or caries seizes the body or bodies of one or more of the vertebrae, it sometimes happens that the particular kind of curvature which makes the subject of these sheets is the consequence.

9. That this curvature, which is always from within outward, is caused by the erosion or destruction of part of the body or bodies of one or more of the vertebrae; by which means that immediately above the distemper, and that immediately below it, are brought nearer to each other than they should be, the body of the patient bends forward, the spine is curved from within outward, and the tuberosity appears behind, occasioned by the protrusion of the spinal processes of the distempered vertebrae. (See Plate.)

10. That according to the degree of carious erosion, and according to the number of vertebrae affected, the curve must be less or greater.

11. That when the attack is made upon the dorsal vertebrae, the sternum and ribs, for want of proper support, necessarily give way, and other deformity, additional to the curve, is thereby produced.

12. That this kind of caries is always confined to the bodies of the vertebrae, seldom or never affecting the articular processes.

13. That without this erosive destruction of the bodies of the vertebrae, there can be no curvature of the kind which I am speaking of; or, in other words, that erosion is the *sine qua non* of this disease; that although there can be no true curve without caries, yet there is, and that not infrequently, caries without curve.

14. That the caries with curvature and useless limbs, is most frequently of the cervical or dorsal vertebrae; the caries without curve, of the lumbal, though this is by no means constant or necessary.

15. That is the case of carious spine, without curvature, it most frequently happens, that internal abscesses and collections of matter are formed, which matter makes its way outward, and appears in the hip, groin, or thigh; or being detained within the body, destroys the patient; the real and immediate cause of whose death is seldom known or even rightly guessed at, unless the dead body be examined.

16. That what are commonly called lumbal and psoas abscesses, are not infrequently induced in this manner, and therefore when we use these terms, we should be understood to mean only a description of the course which such matter has pursued in its way outwards, or the place where it makes its appearance externally, the terms really mean nothing more, nor conveying any precise idea of the nature, seat, or origin of a distemper subject to great variety, and from which variety its very different symptoms and events, in different subjects, can alone be accounted for.

17. That contrary to the general opinion, a caries of the spine is more frequently a cause than an effect of these abscesses.

18. That the true curvature of the spine, from within outward, of which the paralytic, or useless state of the lower limbs, is a too frequent consequence, is itself but *one* effect of a distempered spine; such case being always attended with a number of complaints which arise from the same cause: the generally-received opinion, therefore, that all the attending symptoms are derived from the curvature, considered abstractedly, is by no means founded in truth, and may be productive of very erroneous conduct.

19. That in the case of true curvature, attended with useless limbs, there never is a *dislocation*, properly to be so called, but that the alteration in the figure of the backbone, is caused solely by the erosion, and destruction of a part of one or more of the corpora vertebrarum; and, that as there can be no true curvature without caries, it must be demonstrably clear, that there must have been a distempered state of parts previous to such erosion; from all which it follows, that this distemper, call it by what name you please, ought to be regarded as the original cause of the whole; that is of the caries, of the curvature, and all the attendant mischiefs.

20. That whosoever will consider the real state of the parts when a caries has taken place and the parts surrounding it are in a state of ulceration, must see why none of the attempts by swings, screws, &c., can possibly do any good but on the contrary, if they act so as to produce any effect at all, it must be a bad one.

21. That the discharge, by means of issues produces a cessation of the erosion of the bones; that this is followed by an incarnation of the bones, by means of which the bodies of the vertebrae coalesce and unite with each other forming a kind of anchylosis.

Brodie's Abscess: Sir Benjamin Brodie, 1783-1862

A parson's son, Benjamin Brodie was born at Winterslow, Wiltshire. After studying at Abernethy's School of Anatomy and the Great Windmill School he went to St. George's Hospital as a pupil of Everard Home (who is mainly remembered as the man who plagiarised John Hunter and later burned Hunter's manuscripts to avoid being rumbled). He qualified in 1805 and became Assistant Surgeon at St. George's at the age of 24. This involved a great deal of clinical work, as his chief's appearances were infrequent; further, at this period, out-patient departments were hardly a feature of hospital life.

He became one of the best known surgeons of his day and attended many prominent people including George IV. In 1818 his work on *Diseases of the Joints* appeared—though it does not seem original or fresh today, it was one of the early monographs, and correlated pathological and clinical aspects in a systematic manner with the object of distinguishing between different types of joint disease. In 1843 he introduced the Fellowship examination of the Royal College of Surgeons in an attempt to improve the education and standing of surgeons. In 1858 he was President of the Royal Society and in the same year first President of the General Medical Committee.

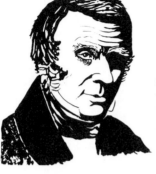

1832

AN ACCOUNT
of
SOME CASES
of
CHRONIC ABSCESSES OF THE TIBIA
by B. C. Brodie, F.R.S.,
and Surgeon to St. George's Hospital

I am not aware that any cases exactly similar to those which I am about to relate have been recorded by authors: and as they appear to me to throw some light on the history and treatment of a rare but very serious disease, I am led to believe that they are not unworthy of being communicated to the Medical and Chirurgical Society.

Case 1

Mr. P. about twenty-four years of age, consulted me in October, 1824, under the following circumstances.

There was a considerable enlargement of the lower extremity of the right tibia, extending to the distance of two or three inches from the ankle-joint. The integuments at this part were tense, and they adhered closely to the surface of the bone.

The patient complained of a constant pain referred to the enlarged bone, and neighbouring parts. The pain was always sufficiently distressing; but he was also liable to more severe paroxysms in which his sufferings were described as most excruciating. These paroxysms recurred at irregular intervals, confining him to his room for many successive days, and being attended with a considerable degree of constitutional disturbance. Mr. P. described the disease as having existed more than twelve years, and as having rendered his life miserable during the whole of that period.

In the course of this time he had been under the care of various surgeons, and various modes of treatment had been resorted to without any permanent advantage. The remedies which I prescribed for him were equally inefficacious. Finding himself without any prospect of being relieved by other means, he made up his mind to lose the limb by amputation; and Mr. Travers having seen him with me in consultation, and having concurred in the opinion, that this was the best course which could be pursued, the operation was performed accordingly.

On examining the amputated limb, it was found that a quantity of new bone had been deposited on the surface of the lower extremity of the tibia. This deposition of new bone was manifestly the result of inflammation of the periosteum at some former period. It was not less than one-third of an inch in thickness, and when the tibia was divided longitudinally with a saw, the line at which the new and old bone were united with each other, was distinctly to be seen.

The whole of the lower extremity of the tibia was harder and more compact than under ordinary circumstances, in consequence, as it appeared, of some deposit of bone in the cancellous structure, and in its centre, about one-third of an inch above the ankle, there was a cavity the size of an ordinary walnut, filled with a dark-coloured pus. The bone immediately surrounding this cavity, was distinguished from that in the neighbourhood by its being of a whiter colour, and of a still harder texture, and the inner surface of the cavity presented an appearance of high vascularity. The ankle-joint was free from disease.

It is evident that if the exact nature of the disease had been understood, and the bone had been perforated with a trephine, so as to allow the pus collected in its interior to escape, a cure would probably have been effected, without the loss of the limb, and with little or no danger to the patient's life. Such, at least, was the opinion which the circumstances of the case led me to form at the time; and I bore them in my mind, in the expectation that at some future period I might have the opportunity of acting on the knowledge which they afforded me for the benefit of another patient.

After the operation the patient suffered a reactionary haemorrhage and became delirious, dying on the fifth day. He goes on to describe two further cases: both he trephined and both healed.

Here is Brodie's operation note of one of these.

A crucial incision was made through the skin, the angles of which were raised so as to expose a part of the bone above the inner ankle, to which the pain was especially referred. A small trephine was then applied, and a circular portion of bone was removed extending into the cancellous structure. Other portions of bone were removed with a narrow chisel. At last about a dram of pus suddenly escaped and rose into the opening made by the trephine and chisel. On further examination a cavity was discovered from which the pus had flowed, capable of admitting the extremity of the finger. The inner surface of this cavity was exquisitely tender; the patient experiencing the most excruciating pain on the gentlest introduction of the probe into it.

From the time of the operation, the peculiar pain from which the patient had previously suffered, was entirely relieved: and it was not long before he was quite restored to health, and able to walk and pursue his occupations without interruption. I have seen him lately, nearly two years from the time of the operation having been performed, and he continues perfectly well.

Tom Smith's Arthritis of Infancy: Sir Thomas Smith, 1833-1909

Born in Kent, and trained at St. Bartholomew's Hospital, Thomas Smith was later a surgeon there and at Great Ormond Street. He was a good and kindly man, who had no wish to write textbooks. He once said "It is the men who don't get the cases who write the books about them".

His description of septic arthritis of infancy was written while an out-patient assistant at St. Bart's. He also described xanthomatosis of bone (Hand-Schüller-Christian disease) in 1865, long before this triumvirate noticed it.

On the Acute Arthritis of Infants: 1874

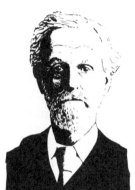

There have come under my observation during the last few years several cases of acute articular disease in infants, which differ so much in their progress and result from any of the recognised joint-affections of childhood, that they seem to me to need what they have not hitherto received, namely, a special description.

The disease to which I propose to direct attention, and which I shall call the *acute arthritis of infants*, probably owes its distinctive features more to the time of life at which it occurs than to any essential difference between it and other recognised joint-affections. It occurs, so far as my experience extends, within the first year of life, and is characterised by the suddenness of its onset and the rapidity of its progress and termination, whether the latter be of a fatal or a favourable kind. It is very dangerous to life, and intensely destructive to the articular ends of the bones, which, of course, at this period of life are largely cartilaginous. Lastly, I would mention as a feature of the disease, that it rarely produces anchylosis, but leaves a child with a limb shortened, by loss of part of the articular end of some bone, and with a weakened, flail-like joint.

I have kept notes of many cases of the disease, twenty-one of which are here reported; they will serve to illustrate its principal characteristics.

The fatal cases here reported, with one or two exceptions, are deficient in one important feature, namely, in the absence of any examination of the viscera. This arises from the fact that most of the infants were out-patients, and that consent to examine the local disease was only obtained on the express condition that the body should not be opened.

The disease which I wish to describe commenced, in all the cases that I have seen, in the first year of life. Eight cases occurred in infants under a month old; four cases in infants under two months; seven cases occurred between the ages of two and six months, and three children were between six months and a year old. In all cases I have to relate, the disease first attacked either the shoulder, hip or knee, and often more than one joint was subsequently affected in the same infant.

The disease was ushered in with restricted movement, and usually flexion of the joint affected, followed by pain, swelling, and rapid suppuration within the joint; the redness of the skin was often but little marked until the abscess was on the point of bursting. After the abscess had opened or had been punctured, if recovery took place, the discharge generally ceased to flow much sooner than is usual in ordinary cases of suppuration within the cavity of a joint. When death occurred, it resulted from exhaustion from local suppuration, or, as one may believe in certain cases, from this, together with a general condition of pyaemia, with secondary affection of internal organs.

On post-mortem examination, I have found in all instances a considerable and rapid loss of substance in the articular end of one of the long bones entering into the joint affected. In some cases this absorption or ulceration has proceeded from the joint surface towards the deeper parts. In others, the destruction of tissue had commenced in abscess within the articular end of the bone, which, after excavating and destroying more or less of the interior of the bone, had burst into the joint by a small opening near the margin of the articular cartilage. In Case III, the existence of subarticular abscess was first *discovered accidentally* in making a section of the bone. I cannot doubt that, in times gone by, when I was unaware of this peculiar pathological condition, I have overlooked many instances of subarticular abscess from neglecting to make a section of the bone in cases of suppuration within joint cavities.*

It seems that in many cases, the formation of a subarticular abscess in the bone must have been the first step in the joint affection, since, while the articular end of the bone was extensively excavated, the aperture through which the abscess had burst into the joint was a mere pin-hole, and though the joint contained pus, the articular cartilage was apparently healthy.

The following case will serve to illustrate the ordinary course of the disease in a well-marked case.

Case I

Arthritis of the Knee in an Infant four weeks old—Extensive Destruction of the Condyloid End of the Femur

I saw Joseph Palmer at the Children's Hospital on March 21, 1866. He was four weeks old, and was the first child of apparently healthy parents. At his birth instruments were used, but no traction by the legs was employed. Four days after birth the left knee was noticed to be permanently flexed, and soon afterward the joint became swollen. When I first saw the child he was very ill, and the knee-joint was distended with pus; the abscess was opened, and a large quantity of matter escaped, and in a few days the child died.

---

* I have given the name subarticular abscess to abscess cavities formed beneath the articular cartilage, either in the cartilaginous or osseous structure of the end of the bone.

On post-mortem examination the knee-joint was found full of pus, the cartilage over the tibia was healthy in appearance, as was also that covering the patella and external condyle of the femur. There was a large ragged hole in the cartilage of the internal condyle, large enough to admit one's finger; this led into a deep excavated cavity in the bone and ossifying cartilage; this cavity occupied a large part of the articular end of the femur, of which little remained but the shell.

2 BONE DISEASE

Paget's Disease of Bone: Sir James Paget, 1814-1899

Paget bears many similarities to Dupuytren—he had a clinico-pathological approach and recognised several conditions for the first time. His descriptions are so full and accurate that they have not been bettered.

He was born in Yarmouth, the son of a brewer and ship-owner of varying fortunes. After he had been apprenticed to the local surgeon for four years, he went to St. Bartholomew's Hospital. As a student he discovered that the little calcific deposits in the muscles of cadavers were due to a parasite, later identified as *Trichina spiralis*. His father's money ran out and he could not afford a surgical dressership. He does not seem to have occupied any surgical post until he was elected a consultant in 1847. He was curator of the museum and a demonstrator in morbid anatomy, supplementing his meagre income as part-time sub-editor of the *London Medical Gazette*.

As a result of these difficulties he was not a brilliant operator but rather a sound clinician and a good orator.

> The popularity of Sir James Paget is unbounded. When it is known that he is to address a meeting, the hall in which he is announced to appear is crowded with an earnest, intelligent audience, which realises that it has come to be instructed and pleased, and that its expectations will not be disappointed. His manner of speaking is entirely free from that drawl and hesitation which are so common to many of his countrymen. So great is his reputation for versatility and for the rapid acquisition of knowledge, that it has been said of him, 'Give him six weeks and he will lecture on Oriental languages'.
>
> Samuel D. Gross (1805-84).

In 1851 he was elected to the Royal Society and became President of the Royal College of Surgeons in 1875. He nearly died in 1871 as a result of an infected cut he suffered whilst carrying out a post mortem—this led to his resignation from Bart's.

Good literary style is seldom found between medical covers: this excerpt from Paget's first paper on Osteitis Deformans is an outstanding example of style. He unfolds the narrative as a story-teller and includes, in no more than a footnote, one of the earliest descriptions of ankylosing spondylitis.

1877

ON A FORM
of
CHRONIC INFLAMMATION OF BONES
(Osteitis deformans)

I hope it will be agreeable to the Society if I make known some of the results of a study of a rare disease of bones.

The patient on whom I was able to study it was a gentleman of good family, whose parents and grandparents lived to old age with apparently sound health, and among whose relatives no disease was known to have prevailed. Especially, gout and rheumatism, I was told, were not known among them; but one of his sisters died with chronic cancer of the breast.

Till 1854, when he was forty-six years old, the patient had no sign of disease, either general or local. He was a tall, thin, well-formed man, father of healthy children, very active in both mind and body. He lived very temperately, could digest, as he said, anything, and slept always soundly.

At forty-six, from no assigned cause, unless it were that he lived in a rather cold and damp place in the North of England, he began to be subject to aching pains in his thighs and legs. They were felt chiefly after active exercise, but were never severe; yet the limbs became less agile or, as he called them "less serviceable", and after about a year he noticed that his left shin was misshapen. His general health, however, was quite unaffected.

I first saw this gentleman in 1856, when these things had been observed for about two years. Except that he was very grey and looked rather old for his age, he might have been considered as in perfect health. He walked with strength and power, but somewhat stiffly. His left tibia, especially in its lower half, was broad, and felt nodular and uneven, as if not only itself but its periosteum and the integuments over it were thickened. In a much less degree similar changes could be felt in the lower half of the left femur. This limb was occasionally but never severely painful, and there was no tenderness of pressure. Every function appeared well discharged, except that the urine showed rather frequent deposits of lithates. Regarding the case as one of chronic periositis, I advised iodide of potassium and Liquor Potassae; but they did no good.

Three years later I saw the patient with Mr. Stanley. He was in the same good general health, but the left tibia had become larger, and had a well-marked anterior curve, as if lengthened while its ends were held in place by their attachments to the unchanged fibula. The left femur also was now distinctly enlarged, and felt tuberous at the junction of its upper and middle thirds, and was arched forwards and outwards, so that he could not bring the left knee into contact with the right. There was also some appearance of widening of the left side of the pelvis, the nates on this side being flattened and lowered, and the great trochanter projecting nearly half an inch further from the middle line. The left limb was about a quarter of an inch shorter than the right. The patient believed that the right side of his skull was enlarged, for his hats had become too tight; but the change was not clearly visible.

Notwithstanding these progressive changes, the patient suffered very little; he had lived actively, walking, riding, and engaging in all the usual pursuits of a country gentleman, and, except that his limb was clumsy, he might have been indifferent to it. He had taken various medicines, but none had done any good, and iodine, in whatever form, had always done harm.

In the next seventeen years of his life I rarely saw him, but the story of his disease, of which I often heard, may be briefly told and with few dates, for its progress was nearly uniform and very slow. The left femur and tibia became larger, heavier, and somewhat more curved. Very slowly those of the right limb followed the same course, till they gained very nearly the same size and shape. The limbs thus became nearly symmetrical in their deformity, the curving of the left being only a little more outward than that of the right. At the same time, or later, the knees became gradually bent, and, as if by rigidity of their fibrous tissues, lost much of their natural range and movement.

The skull became gradually larger, so that nearly every year, for many years, his hat, and the helmet that he wore as a member of a Yeomanry Corps, needed to be enlarged. In 1844 he wore a shako measuring twenty-two and a half inches inside; in 1876 his hat measured twenty-seven and a quarter inches inside. In its enlargement, however, the head retained its natural shape and, to the last, looked intellectual, though with some exaggeration.

The changes of shape and size in both the limbs and the head were arrested, or increased only imperceptibly, in the last three or four years of life.

The spine very slowly became curved and almost rigid. The whole of the cervical vertebrae and the upper dorsal formed a strong posterior, not angular, curve; and an anterior curve, of similar shape, was formed by the lower dorsal and lumbar vertebrae. The length of the spine thus seemed lessened, and from a height of six feet one inch he sank to about five feet nine inches. At the same the chest became contracted, narrow, flattened laterally, deep from before backwards, and the movements of the ribs and of the spine were lessened. There was no complete rigidity, as if by union of bones, but all the movements were very restrained, as if by shortening and rigidity of the fibrous connections of the vertebrae and ribs.

The shape and habitual posture of the patient were thus made strange and peculiar. His head was advanced and lowered, so that the neck was very short, and the chin, when he held his head at ease, was more than an inch lower than the top of the sternum.

The short narrow chest suddenly widened into a much shorter and broader abdomen, and the pelvis was wide and low. The arms appeared unnaturally long, and, though the shoulders were very high, the hands hung low down by the thighs and in front of them.

Altogether, the attitude in standing looked simian, strangely in contrast with the large head and handsome features.*

All changes of shape and attitude are well shown in sketches from photographs taken six months before death. Only the lowering of the necks of the femora is not shown. In measurement after death the axes of the shaft and neck of the right femur formed an angle of only 100 degrees instead of 120 degrees or 125 degrees, and this change of shape added to the appearance of increased width of the pelvis.

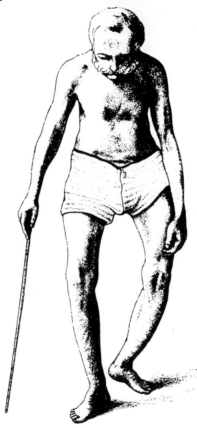

Paget's Disease

But with all these changes in shape and mobility of the head, spine, and lower limbs, the upper limbs remained perfect, and there was no disturbance of the general health.

In 1870, when the disease had existed sixteen years, the left knee joint was, for a time, actively inflamed and its cavity was distended with fluid. But the inflammation soon subsided, only leaving the joint stiffer and more bent.

About this time some signs of insufficiency of the mitral valve were observed, but the patient now lived so quietly, and moved with so little speed, that this defect gave him no considerable distress.

In December, 1872, sight was partially destroyed by retinal haemorrhage, first in one eye, then in the other, and at nearly the same time he began to be somewhat deaf. In the summer of 1874 he had frequent cramps in the legs, and neuralgic pains, which were described as "jumping over all the upper part of the body except the head", but change of air seemed to cure them.

In January, 1876, he began to complain of pain in his left forearm and elbow which, at first, was thought to be neuralgic. But it grew worse, and swelling appeared about the upper third of the radius and increased rapidly, so that, when I saw him in the middle of February, it seemed certain that a firm medullary or osteoid cancerous growth was forming round the radius.

---

* An attitude somewhat similar is given by a rare form of what I suppose to be general chronic rheumatoid arthritis of the spine involving its articulations with the ribs. The spine droops and is stiff, the chest is narrow, the ribs scarcely move, the abdomen, is low and broad, but there is no deformity of head or limbs.

Still, the general health was good. Auscultation could detect mitral disease, but the appetite and the digestion were unimpaired, the urine was healthy, the mind as clear, patient, and calm as ever. As letters about him at this time said "his general health has been excellent"; "he is free from pain except in the left arm; he sleeps well, enjoys himself, and does not know what a headache is".

After this time, however, together with rapid increase of the growth upon the radius, there were gradual failure of strength and emaciation, and on the 24th March, after two days of distress with pleural effusion on the right side, he died.

The body was examined five days after death, and showed no marked signs of decomposition. As it lay on a flat board its posture was remarkable, for the head was upraised to the level of the sternum, being supported by the rigid and arched spine, and the lower limbs, with the knees bent and stiff, rested on the heels and nates.

The right pleural cavity contained at least a pint of pale serous fluid, with flakes and strings of inflammatory exudation. The lung was compressed, and in its pleural covering were numerous small nodular masses of pale cancerous substance. The proper pulmonary structure appeared healthy, and so did the left lung and its pleura, except that in the pleura and anterior mediastinum there were many small masses of cancer.

The heart was enlarged but thin-walled. The tricuspid and pulmonary valves and artery were healthy; the mitral valve was opaque, contracted, stiffened with atheromatous and calcareous deposits.

In the bones of the skeleton, except the left radius, no signs of disease appeared externally, but I regret that they were not all more carefully examined, for I think that, at least in the clavicles and pelvis, some changes like those in the long bones of the lower limbs would have been found.

The upper third of the left radius was involved in a large ovoid mass of pale grey and white soft cancerous substance, similar to that of the nodules in the pleurae and mediastinum, but with growths of bone extending into it. The rest of the radius and the ulna appeared quite healthy.

Some nodules of similar cancerous substance were imbedded in the bones of the vault of the skull.

The curvatures of the spine and its rigidity appeared due to shortening and hardening of fibrous structures. The vertebrae appeared healthy; there was no appearance of overgrowth or anchylosis among them.

In no part, whether near or far from the diseased bones, was there an indication of any change of structure in skin, muscle, tendon, or fascia; but in the right hip-joint and in the left knee-joint there was some thinning and wasting of articular cartilage, such as one sees in chronic rheumatic arthritis. The other hip- and knee-joints and both ankle-joints were healthy.

23

In the arteries of the lower limbs there was extensive atheromatous and calcareous degeneration.

The conditions of all the long bones were so similar that one description may serve for the altered structure of both femora and tibiae.

The periosteum was not visibly changed, not thicker or more than usually adherent.

The outer surface of the walls of the bones was irregularly and finely nodular, as with external deposits or outgrowths of bone, deeply grooved with channels for the large periosteal blood-vessels, finely but visibly perforated in every part for transmission of the enlarged small vessels. Everything seemed to indicate a greatly increased quantity of blood in the vessels of the bone.

The medullary structures appeared to the naked eye as little changed as the periosteum. The medullary spaces were filled with soft, yellow, ruddy, and bright crimson medulla, of apparently healthy consistence. The medullary laminae and cancelli had a normal aspect and arrangement, and in the shafts of the long bones the medullary spaces were not encroached upon.

The compact substance of the bones was, in every part, increased in thickness.

The thickening of the walls of the shafts of the bones appeared due chiefly to outward expansion and some superficial outgrowth. In some places there were faint appearances of separation of parts of the outer layers of the walls, and of these becoming thick and porous, while the corresponding parts of the inner layers were less changed; but in the greater part of the walls the whole construction of the bone was altered into a hard, porous or finely reticulate substance, like very fine coral. In some places, especially in the walls of the femur, there were small, ill-defined patches of pale, dense, and hard bone looking as solid as brick.

In the compact covering of the articular ends of the long bones, and in those of the neck and great trochanter of the femur, and in the patellae the increase of thickness was due to encroachment on the cancellous texture, as if by filling of its spaces with compact porous, new-formed bone.

Holding then the disease to be an inflammation of the bones, I would suggest that, for brief reference and for the present, it may be called after its most striking character, osteitis deformans. A better name may be given when more is known of it.

Dyschondroplasia: Louis Ollier, 1830-1900

Ollier was one of the great men of orthopaedics. He devoted his life to his work; in addition to several important clinical papers he carried out research on normal and pathological bone growth considering it not only as a structure but also as a tissue.

He was born at Vans in Ardèche and studied at Lyons and Montpellier. At the age of 30 he became senior surgeon at Lyons. In the 1870 war he was a battle surgeon, looking after the wounded of both sides. In 1894 he was decorated with the Order of Knight of the Legion of Honour by the French President. A few hours after the ceremony the President was assassinated and Ollier was called to him, but his injuries were too severe for Ollier to be able to save his life.

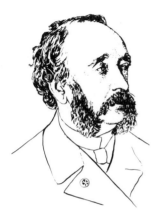

Dyschondroplasia: Ollier's Disease, 1899

M. Ollier described under this name a new type of disease which he has been able to determine by means of clinical observation and radiography. It consists of the irregular formation and development of cartilaginous tissues which have a tendency to delayed ossification.

This differentiates it from the chondroplasia of Parrot, in which there is atrophy or lack of development of the bone and brings it closer to multiple osteogenic exostoses.

The first case observed by M. Ollier in June, 1897, was a little girl of $6\frac{1}{2}$ who presented with an inturned forearm and femur, exostoses of the femur of a cartilaginous appearance, and deformities of the fingers, which were shorter, thicker and soft on pressure. Radiography showed a series of irregular spaces that were radiotranslucent and cartilaginous in the diaphyses of the phalanges.

A little later M. Ollier observed an analagous case in a young girl of 9. The femora were curved in; the upper end of the fibula, which was slightly atrophic, carried a mass resembling cartilage. Radiographs of the fingers presented the same abnormal appearance of cartilaginous spaces in the phalanges.

Since then, M. Destot has seen and radiographed a third case. The disease appeared to have been present for a long time, developing without pain, with a tendency to delayed ossification, and the persistence of the initial deformities. This affection does not resemble osteomalacia, nor rickets, nor the chondromata which have no tendency to ossification. There is a need for further observation to define its place; but it appears to M. Ollier to be a completely new disease entity, which must be given a new name, that of Dyschondroplasia.

In the discussion which followed the presentation of his paper, Ollier put forward the view that the difference between dyschondroplasia and osteogenic exostoses was 'a difference of form and situation, but not of nature'. He hoped that it might eventually be possible to treat the cases by stimulating the cartilage to ossify.

Melorheostosis: Andre Léri, 1875-1930

Léri was a follower of the followers of Charcot. His interests were catholic because specialisation was anathema to him. He achieved distinction as a neurologist, opthalmologist, psychiatrist and orthopaedic physician.

After a doctoral thesis on ocular manifestations of tabes, he joined Marie to expand Marie's original account of ankylosing spondylitis. He described the neurological manifestations of spina bifida occulta, and recognised that osteo-arthritis of the spine could cause root pain.

He recognised and named two rare diseases of bone—pleonosteosis in 1921 and melorheostosis in 1922. He wrote a book on vertebral disease in 1926.

An undescribed Condition of Bone: Flowing Hyperostosis along the Entire Length of a Limb or Melorheostosis: by Andre Léri and Joanny 1922

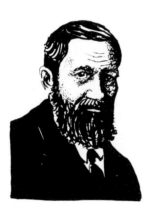

The patient that we are presenting is suffering from a bone condition which we have not found mentioned in medical literature. It consists of an unusual hyperostosis stretching right up the bones of one upper limb, and limited to that limb only:

Mme B. is 39. At the age of 10 she had noticed a deformity of the fingers, characterised by a slight separation of the tips of the index and middle fingers of the left hand. At 17 she had a fall on the left elbow, and it was after this fall that she had found it impossible to extend the elbow fully.

The abnormal development of the bones of this limb had occurred slowly, progressively, without ever bothering her, and without any pain up to the age of 35. In 1918, she woke one morning with pains in her left shoulder and left elbow, accompanied by impaired function: for three days she was unable to do her hair or dress herself, then mobility returned. The pain, however, persisted, though it was less intense, and rather vague, consisting more of feelings of numbness than of real pain, and was most noticeable at night.

She came to consult us for the functional impairment of the elbow, the painful feelings in the arm, and the deformity of the fingers.

On examination, what struck us first of all was the deformity and hypertrophy of the index and middle fingers of the left hand. These two fingers were huge, and seemed to belong to quite another hand compared with the neighbouring fingers; they recalled certain congenital macrodactylies. We also noticed that they were no longer than the other fingers, but their circumference was considerably greater. Furthermore, far from being straight, they showed a series of hard lumps, about the size of a small nut, pressing up under the skin, but not adhering to it. The index and middle finger forked away from each other at the level of the middle phalanx, the middle finger curved outwards—the ends of the fingers were two centimetres apart. The index and middle fingers had normal extension, but flexion was very limited, particularly of the index finger. On examining these enlarged fingers, which were bumpy along the lengths of the bones (but not at the joints), and were hard, and rather stiff, one had the impression of a case of multiple chondromata of the hand.

But, beside this, we found deformity and limited movement of all other parts of the upper left limb.

The carpal and metacarpal bones of the left hand, in the line of the 2nd and 3rd metacarpals, formed a hard, elongated protuberance over which the skin was stretched. Extension of the wrist was very slightly reduced by comparison with the healthy side; flexion, however, was much reduced—50° instead of 90°.

Palpation of the left forearm revealed nothing abnormal; but the movements of the elbow were extremely limited, the elbow permanently remained flexed to almost a right angle, active and passive movements were from 80° of flexion to 110° of extension; supination was good, but pronation was very restricted.

Palpation of the left arm revealed a thickened humerus, clearly larger than that on the other side, but because of the intervening muscle mass it was difficult to say whether it was regular or irregular. The coracoid apophysis was obviously thickened. Shoulder movements were grossly diminished—rotation was absent, abduction and flexion did not exceed 35° to 40°, extension alone was normal.

These combined findings no longer resemble chondromata of the hand, but rather make one think of some affection similar to Ollier's dyschondroplasia.

Radiographs show that it is something completely different; the bony thickenings are not at all cartilaginous; they are *osseous* and in fact composed of very thick and compact bone.

The three phalanges of the index and middle fingers and the corresponding metacarpals are very hyperostotic and formed of a very opaque bone, most irregularly indented on the surface, and possessing nothing like the regular contours of normal bone. One thing should be noticed—the lateral side of the first phalanx and the metacarpal of the middle finger have escaped the hyperostosis.

At the wrist, only the trapezoid, os magnum, and lunate are thickened, to continue the "line of hyperostosis" of the second and third fingers and metacarpals.

In the forearm, it is the lateral edge of the ulna in its lower two-thirds, the medial border of the radius in its upper one-third which have become hyperostotic, thick, and irregular, as if a line of hyperostosis extended from the lunate to the lateral border of the ulna and from there on to the medial border of the radius. The head of the radius is thickened and osteophytic.

In the arm, the humerus is thickened along its length, especially in its lower 2/3 or 3/4, and has widely and irregularly distributed dribbles along its anterior surface. The head of the humerus, the glenoid, and the coracoid apophysis are widely flecked with streaks of very dense bone.

We found nothing else abnormal; the opposite limb, in particular, was completely normal.

Thus, we found, throughout the entire length of the left upper limb of this patient, a most unusual bone hypertrophy—not occupying all the bones, nor all of one bone but only certain bones and certain parts of these bones. In this apparent irregularity of its distribution, there is, nevertheless, something remarkably regular—the trail of hyperostosis, which seems to continue on the X-ray almost in a straight line, leaving intact the parts of the neighbouring bones which adjoin it.

This hyperostosis is essentially irregular at its margins—dribbling, so to speak—so that one has radiographically, the impression of candle wax drippings along the bones from the shoulder to the extremities of the second and third fingers.

Furthermore this is clearly a question of hyperostosis and not of periostitis, as X-rays patently demonstrate that different layers of bone are involved.

This hyperostotic candle drip does not follow the distribution of any peripheral nerve, nerve root or nerve tract; X-ray of the spinal column has been carried out and showed nothing abnormal. In addition, there did not appear to be any connection between the form of the drips and the distribution of the vessels. Syphilis did not appear to be the cause; we found no history or sign of this; the W.R. was negative, and although she had had two miscarriages she had also had two children aged 18 and 14 who are very healthy. Moreover, since the history of this complaint goes back to the age of ten, one would think of some hereditary element—but we found nothing in her family history—her mother is alive and well, her father died at the age of 65 from arterio-sclerosis. The lesions had no resemblance to syphylitic osteitis, neither in their evolution nor in their local appearance (thick seams instead of relatively regular periostitis), or in their distribution.

No osteodystrophy so far known has this appearance or distribution.

We have been tempted to consider this a simple fault of bone development, or of the process of ossification recognising that the cause of its unusual appearance still completely escapes us.

We think one may call the disease "Melorheostosis", a term which leaves in suspense all problems of pathogenesis and aetiology, but which indicates the essential clinical characteristics—flowing hyperostosis occupying the length of a limb.

In 1928 he described eight further cases affecting the upper limb, and in 1930 when a further case presented itself, he biopsied a metacarpal. The bone had the colour and consistency of ivory. Histologically it was simply very dense bone; culture was negative. He wondered whether perhaps a parasite was causing the condition.

Subungual Exostosis: Baron Guillaume Dupuytren, 1777-1835

The "Brigande of the Hôtel Dieu" was born in Central France. The son of a poor advocate, he was kidnapped as a boy by a rich lady from Toulouse on account of his good looks, and, after reclamation, was taken to Paris and educated by a rich cavalry officer. As a medical student he endured poverty, allegedly reading books by the light of oil prepared from dissecting cadavers. He became Surgeon-in-chief at the Hôtel Dieu at the age of 36, and worked tremendously hard at teaching, operating and seeing 10,000 private patients a year. He became very rich, and was probably a most unpleasant person to meet, but his writings are delightful to read for their lucid, accurate descriptions and deductive reasoning. Like many of those who are mentioned here, he combined accurate clinical observation with a tremendous interest in pathology. His works are easily readable, very informative and he is quoted in this collection more than any other author.

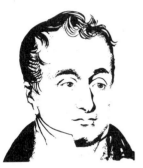

Subungual Exostosis: Dupuytren, 1817

Case 5

Exostosis on the Ungual Phalanx of the Great Toe: *Extirpation and Cure* Louise Cassin, a laundress, aged 20, was admitted into the Hôtel Dieu in 1817, with an osseous tumour, about the size of a large pea, on the outer border of the last phalanx of the great toe; the nail had grown into the back part of it, and occasioned pain. This morbid growth was removed with a bistoury, and the wound was afterwards cauterized; portions of the nail and necrosed bone afterwards exfoliated, and the patient quitted the hospital before she was quite well. This excrescence likewise presented an osseous nucleus.

The above affection has not been noticed, as far as I know, by any author. It is painful and inconvenient rather than dangerous; and its characteristics are such as the details of the above cases exhibit. I know not what cause to ascribe it to, for it usually occurs in individuals who have received no injury, and is apparently unassociated with a scrofulous disthesis or syphilitic taint. The morbid growth in question has been usually mistaken for a wart, and treated as such by cauteries, which are always, under these circumstances, productive of much mischief. The nail has in other cases been fixed upon as the seat of the disease, and removed accordingly, with, I need scarcely add, no beneficial effect. The structure of the excrescence is such as I have already described: it usually yields to the knife, but in some instances requires stronger instruments for its removal. If allowed to proceed, intractable ulceration ensues; and in one case of this sort I saw the ungual phalanx of the great toe removed entirely for this affection. In performing the operation, it may be occasionally necessary to cut away the nail, but this is usually uncalled for: care should be taken to extirpate the whole of the diseased growth, or it will be reproduced. It has fallen to my lot to operate on as many as thirty cases such as I have just described.

3 JOINT DISEASE

Internal Derangement of the Knee: William Hey, 1736-1819

William Hey was the founder of surgery at Leeds and initiated the construction of a hospital there. His life story was written by his pupil, John Pearson; it is a most remarkable work, describing his lofty ideals and religious fervour, so much so that it resembles a book about a saint destined for Sunday reading by a Victorian family. Many consultants would envy this devotion from a pupil.

He was born in Pudsey near Leeds, and his father was a dry-salter (a dealer in the ingredients for manufacturing cloth). At the age of 14 he was apprenticed to a surgeon and apothecary and nearly died of an overdose of opium whilst studying its effects. In 1757 he went to St. George's and when he qualified set up in practice in Leeds. He was a busy general surgeon and accoucheur and a friend of Joseph Priestly, the physicist, who proposed him as an F.R.S. in 1775. Hey was always a fervent churchman: he preached to Wesley and wrote tracts. During his time as Mayor and Magistrate at Leeds he enforced the Sunday Observance Laws very strictly. The local inhabitants retaliated by burning an effigy of him.

He wrote a small book on surgery which includes several chapters on orthopaedics. He described subacute osteomyelitis of the tibia before Brodie and advocated deroofing the lesion. His interest in the knee may be due to the fact that he banged his knee getting out of a bath in 1773, and remained lame all his days. However he coined the phrase 'internal derangement of the knee', and described meniscus injuries. He wrote about loose bodies and introduced tarso-metatarsal amputation.

He died in 1819, and his son succeeded him as surgeon at Leeds Infirmary.

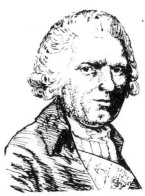

On Internal Derangement of the Knee Joint: William Hey, 1803

The joint of the knee is so firmly supported on all sides by tendinous ligamentous substances that the bones of the thigh and leg are very rarely separated from each other, so as to form a *dislocation*, in the common sense of the term. Great violence must take place, and a considerable laceration must happen, before the tibia can be completely separated from the os femoris. Yet this joint is not unfrequently affected with an internal derangement of its component parts; and that sometimes in consequence of trifling accidents. The disease is, indeed, now and then removed, as suddenly as it is produced, by the natural motions of the joint, without surgical assistance; but it may remain for weeks or months; and will then become a serious misfortune, as it causes a considerable degree of lameness. I am not acquainted with any author who has described either the disease or the remedy; I shall, therefore, give such a description as my own experience has furnished me with, and such as will suffice to distinguish a complaint, which, when recent, admits of an easy method of cure.

This disorder may happen either with, or without, contusion. In the latter case it is readily distinguished. In the former, the symptoms are equivocal, till the effects of the contusion are removed. When no contusion has happened, or the effects of it are removed, the joint, with respect to its shape, appears to be uninjured. If there is any difference from its usual appearance, it is, that the ligament of the patella appears rather more relaxed than in the sound limb. The leg is readily bent or extended by the hands of the surgeon, and without pain to the patient; at most, the degree of uneasiness caused by this flexion and extension is trifling. But the patient himself cannot freely bend, nor perfectly extend, the limb in walking; he is compelled to walk with an invariable and small degree of flexion. Though the patient is obliged to keep the leg thus stiff in walking; yet in sitting down the affected joint will move like the other.

The complaint which I have described may be brought on, I apprehend, by any such alteration in the state of the joint, as will prevent the condyles of the os femoris from moving truly in the hollow formed by the semilunar cartilages and articular depressions of the tibia. An unequal tension of the lateral, or cross ligaments, of the joint, or some slight derangement of the semilunar cartilages, may probably be sufficient to bring on the complaint. When the disorder is the effect of contusion, it is most likely that the lateral ligament on one side of the joint may be rendered somewhat more rigid than usual; and hereby prevent that equable motion of the condyles of the os femoris, which is necessary for walking with firmness.

The method of cure, which I am about to propose, must not be used while there is any inflammatory affection, or swelling of the joint; but only when these effects of contusion are removed. The following cases will further illustrate the nature of this complaint; and point out the method which I have hitherto found successful in removing it.

Case 2

In 1784, the honourable Miss Harriet Ingram (now Mrs. Ashton), as she was playing with a child, and making a considerable exertion, in stretching herself forwards, and stooping to take hold of the child, while she rested upon one leg, brought on an immediate lameness in the knee joint of that leg on which she stood. The disorder was considered as a simple sprain; and a plaster was applied round the joint. As the lameness did not diminish in the course of five or six days, I was desired to visit her.

Upon comparing the knee, I could perceive no difference, except that, when the limbs were placed in a state of complete extension, the ligament of the patella of the injured joint seemed to be rather more relaxed, than in that joint which had received no injury. When I moved the affected knee by a gentle flexion and extension, my patient complained of no pain; yet she could not perfectly extend the leg in walking, nor bend it in raising the foot from the floor; but moved as if the joint had been stiff, limping very much, and walking with pain.

I thought it probable, that the sudden exertion might in some degree have altered the situation of the crossed ligaments, or otherwise have displaced the condyles of the os femoris with respect to the semilunar cartilages, so that the condyles might meet with some resistance when the flexor or extensor muscles were put into action, and thereby the free motion of the joint might be hindered, when the incumbent weight of the body pressed the thigh bone closely against the tibia; though this derangement was not so great as to prevent the joint, when relaxed, from being moved with ease.

To remedy this derangement, I placed my patient upon an elevated seat, which had nothing underneath it that could prevent the leg from being pushed backward towards the posterior part of the thigh. I then extended the joint by the assistance of one hand placed just above the knee, while with the other hand I grasped the leg. During the continuance of the extension I suddenly moved the leg backwards, that it might make as acute an angle with the thigh as possible. This operation I repeated once, and then desired the young lady to try how she could walk. Whatever may be thought of my theory, my practice proved successful; for she was immediately able to walk without lameness, and on the third day after this reduction she danced at a private ball without inconvenience, or receiving any injury from the exercise.

Baker's Cyst: William Morrant Baker, 1839-1896

Born at Andover, the son of a solicitor, William Baker, after being apprenticed to a local surgeon, studied at St. Bartholomew's Hospital. He was a very mature student; he passed the Fellowship at the age of 25, and married the anaesthetist's sister, but he did not get on to the staff as a full surgeon until the age of 43. He passed the intervening years as Casualty Surgeon, assistant to Out-Patients and assistant to Paget in private practice. At one time he was in charge of the skin department, and was for a long while an anatomy lecturer.

He was a general surgeon, who entered the era of antiseptic surgery without being attracted to it, and was regarded as a good opinion rather than a good operator. He wrote widely on general surgery and examined for several boards; rubber tracheostomy tubes were his invention and he is immortalised by his two papers on synovial cysts.

He retired before his time on account of locomotor ataxy which led to his death.

Baker's Cyst: 1877 & 1885

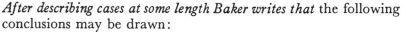

The Formation of Abnormal Synovial Cysts in Connection with the Joints
by W. Morrant Baker

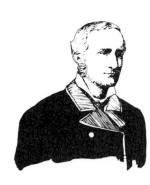

After describing cases at some length Baker writes that the following conclusions may be drawn:

1. That abnormal synovial cysts may be formed in connection, not only with the knee, but in connection with the shoulder, the elbow, the wrist, the hip, and the ankle joints.

2. That the manner of formation of these synovial cysts probably resembles that which has been proved to occur in connection with the knee-joint, namely, that the synovial fluid on reaching a certain amount of tension by accumulation within the joint, finds its way out in the direction of least resistance, either by the channel by which some normal bursa communicates with the joint, or, in the absence of any such channel, by forming first a hernia of the synovial membrane. In both cases, should the tension continue or increase, the fluid at length escapes from the sac, and its boundaries are then formed only by the muscles and other tissues between and amongst which it accumulates.

3. That in the case of the shoulder-joint the abnormal synovial cyst may be found either in front a little below the clavicle, or in the upper arm in the region of the biceps muscle.

4. That in connection with the elbow-joint the cyst is usually placed on the inner side, a little above the internal condyle of the humerus.

5. That in the case of the wrist-joint the synovial cyst may be either in front or behind.

6. In the only case in connection with the hip of which a note has been preserved, the swelling was in the upper part of Scarpa's triangle.

7. In the one case in connection with the ankle-joint the synovial cyst was in front and to the outer side.

8. That the apparent want of direct communication between the joint and the abnormal synovial cyst is frequently deceptive, and should not lead to the inference that no such communication exists.

9. That the caution given in the previous communication, not to interfere by operation with these synovial sacs without good reason, has been justified by increased experience.

Hitherto I have not discovered any relationship between the form of osteo-arthritis with which some of these synovial cysts are associated and locomotor ataxy, but I suspect that in some of them a relationship will be found to exist.

Hoffa's Disease of the Fat Pad of the Knee: Albert Hoffa, 1859-1908

Born in the Cape of Good Hope, South Africa, the son of a German physician, Albert Hoffa was educated in Germany. After qualifying, he established the first private orthopaedic unit in Germany, situated in Würzburg, Bavaria.

He became very well known, wrote and taught a great deal, and founded journals. In 1902 he followed Julius Wolff (known for Wolff's law) as professor at Berlin. Clearly a great and popular man, it is inappropriate that his name should be attached to such a trivial and often unconvincing complaint as hypertrophy of the fat pad of the knee.

Hoffa's Disease: 1904

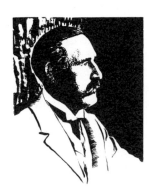

THE INFLUENCE OF THE ADIPOSE TISSUE
WITH REGARD TO THE PATHOLOGY
OF THE KNEE JOINT
A. Hoffa, M.D., Berlin

I first came across this hyperplasia of the fat tissue some years ago on incising a knee-joint for the sake of extirpating the detached meniscus, as I thought, which, however, was intact, and subsequently a great many similar cases were diagnosed by me beforehand showing this hyperplasia of the fat tissue beneath the ligamentum patellae quite typical.

The sound knee joint presents the following anatomic conditions: Under the ligamentum patellae the synovial membrane shows two plicae alares and a plica synovialis patellaris. The former consist of fat tissue with a coating from the synovialis, which stretches from the front margin of the tibia like a fat lobule into the joint, and even sideways beyond the ligamentum patellae. From the central summit of the plica alaris originates the plica synovialis, which is composed of fibrous fat tissue inserted at the fossa intercondyloidae. A sagittal section of the knee joint shows this fatty tissue situated like a wedge between the patella, femur and tibia. While the upper part adheres to the ligamentum patellae, the lower is separated from it by the intervening bursa infrapatellaris profunda and joins the meniscus, also being connected to the periosteum of the front part of the tibia. I have dissected a large number of normal knee joints and always found the above conditions from early childhood upward, the growth of the adipose tissue varying individually, sometimes cachectic individuals showing a larger growth than fat persons.

A section of this fat tissue shows an extensive delicate network of fibrous strings interspersed with fat lobules, the surface being covered with a single layer of endothelial cells and small villi, increasing in number from the central parts toward the surface. These villi consist of a delicate fibrous tissue covered with endothelial cells showing slight vascularity.

This normal adipose tissue is liable to grow and to produce a hyperplasia inflammatoria, even after slight trauma of the knee joint occurring chronically, and can then be felt as a pretty hard mass of fat on both sides of the ligamentum patellae, similar to a lipoma. These growths, I found, differ widely from the normal adipose tissue as regards size, color and solidity.

The growths that I have removed have often been larger than an egg, and, beside the normal color, they show a reddish-yellow tinge, indicating haemorrhages. I have also come across regular blood clots enclosing the above-mentioned villi when the operation was performed immediately after severe attacks of pain. The adipose tissue is much more solid than you usually find it on account of the strong fibrous tissue. A section shows very markedly a network of these solid strings enclosing the enlarged lumina of blood vessels.

This process is characteristic of an inflammatory hyperplasia of the adipose tissue interspersed with strong fibrous strings, and is generally caused by some trauma, either a fall on the knee or some other hurt, such as a sudden jerk, etc. The haemorrhage must be considered as primary, followed by inflammation and exuberant growth of the villi, which are liable to be crushed between the tibia and femur, and this strangulation of the villi regularly makes the patient consult the doctor, showing symptoms quite similar to those of floating bodies of the joint.

The pain is felt quite suddenly on the median side of the joint; the knee can either not be bent or the patient is not able to stretch it. Haemorrhage into the joint itself may have taken place, but this is not generally the case. After a time an atrophy of the quadriceps muscle is more or less developed, and there is a typical swelling of the knee-joint on both sides of the patella, especially in its lower part, where the ligamentum patellae insert, which is often raised by this growth, showing pseudofluctuation. The patient should be examined standing and both knees compared. There is no discharge into the joint, whose power of motion is generally unimpaired, only presenting a slight crepitation, very different from that of arthritis.

DIAGNOSIS

The diagnosis of these cases is not difficult, and they can be separated from the cases of dérangement interne, of separation of the meniscus or of floating bodies. Separation of the meniscus causes the patient to localise the pain exactly within the joint cleft; floating bodies may be determined by Röntgen rays, while in our cases there is perhaps just a slight indication of a shadow within the otherwise clear space between patella, femur and tibia. In all my twenty-one cases which I have observed within the last year and a half, except the first, where a separation of the meniscus was diagnosed, I was able to confirm the diagnosis made beforehand by a subsequent operation.

TREATMENT

Operations on these cases should be undertaken after the other methods, such as massage, compression, etc., have been used without success, by an incision on the median side of the patella. Of course, asepsis is a *conditio sine qua non*, and I have always followed König's "golden rule", to avoid bringing my fingers into contact with the joint and only to work with as few sterilised instruments as possible.

The result is generally very satisfactory, as the disturbance caused by the growths is removed, together with their extirpation, and the operation, carried out under the necessary aseptic conditions, is without danger.

For the first twenty-four hours after the operation I mostly use a small sterilised gauze strip as a drain to the joint. After eight days the sutures are removed and the patients may walk about, movements and massage being soon applied. The full use of the legs is secured in from six to eight weeks.

I can certainly recommend this operation, especially in such cases where other appliances have been resorted to in vain, and I have been able to remove very severe symptoms and definitely heal my patients by this method.

Madelung's Deformity: Otto Madelung, 1846-1926

Madelung was an abdominal surgeon—he flourished during the time that surgery was beginning to have something to offer the patient with abdominal disease. His orthopaedic contributions, though they caused his name to decorate textbooks, were slight.

He was born in Gotha, the son of a merchant, and he studied at Bonn and Tubingen. After serving in the Franco-Prussian war of 1871 he settled in Bonn, and during this time he wrote his paper on wrist deformity. He became Assistant Professor of Surgery at Bonn in 1881, then at Rostock before becoming Professor at Strasburg in 1894, where he was the youngest member of the Medical Faculty. He built up the hospital at Strasburg along German lines and continued to work there until the city was recovered by the French at the end of the First World War. Then all the German Professors were replaced by French and after a period under house arrest he retired to Gottingen.

Apart from his work on intestinal resections, intestinal typhoid, obstruction and so on, he was one of the first advocates of early laparotomy for abdominal injuries. In 1909 he described arthrotomy of the shoulder from behind. His description of deformity at the wrist was not original, and only a little more complete than descriptions by Dupuytren and R. W. Smith which had appeared many years previously.

It is difficult to give much impression of his personality—someone described him as a "serious and conscientious man with a powerful will" and this rather stern picture is supported by one of his sayings: "Every clinical lesson must be prepared and conducted in such a way that every student who contemplates missing the class must feel that he would miss something important".

Spontaneous Anterior Subluxation of the Hand: 1878

Otto Madelung

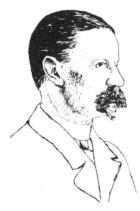

The deformity is most noticeable looking at the subluxation from the ulnar side. The forearm is apparently normally formed. The distal end of the ulna is distinct under the normal though rather tense skin and the styloid process and articular surface can be recognised with the eye and encircled by the finger. The hand viewed on its own is normal but has dropped forwards. The diameter of the wrist is almost twice the normal.

The hand, viewed from the radial side, is less obviously displaced forwards. The extensor tendons, which pass over the radius towards the dorsum of the hand, bridge and obscure the step that was so noticeable on the ulnar side. The antero-posterior diameter appears to be almost doubled. When the distal end of the radius is palpated with the hand dorsiflexed, i.e. with the extensor tendons relaxed, a large portion of the articular surface of the radius may be palpated. At the same time it is noticeable that the posterior lip of the lower end of the radius, which is normally rather sharp, has become more obtuse. If it is compared with the radius of the healthy side it is noticed that the whole distal epiphysis of the radius is angulated volarwards. In some cases, when the hand is inspected in the neutral position between flexion and extension, there is slight deviation of the hand radially and sometimes laterally. Viewed anteriorly the bridge-like prominence of the flexor tendons, particularly flexor carpi radialis, flexor carpi ulnaris, and palmaris longus, becomes noticeable.

Madelung regarded the condition as a defect of growth of the wrist joint. It was not due to trauma or infection. Heavy work by young people produced more pressure on the anterior part of the distal radial epiphysis than the posterior part. In those with "primary weakness of bone" this degree of pressure may cause the anterior part of the epiphysis to stop growing. As a result the lower end of the radius comes to be angulated forwards. The carpal bones are also compressed and show changes.

Treatment was not successful. Surgically replaced hands relapsed. However, Madelung noted that the pain disappeared after a time even when the subluxation was gross, and that the capacity for work was not impaired.

Still's Disease: Sir George Still, 1868-1941

Still was born at Holloway, the son of a surveyor of Customs, and after taking a first in Classics at Cambridge, trained at Guy's. He went to work at the Hospital for Sick Children and remained there all his life.

He quickly became successful because of two good pieces of work written while he was young: he described the disease known after him, and recognised the organism of basal meningitis. He became *the* children's physician of his age. Outwardly he was industrious, distant and impersonal in his dealings with adults; with children he was relaxed and placating.

In addition to writing a standard textbook, he wrote a scholarly "Anthology of Paediatrics", in which he reviewed the history of child care with such penetration and grace that the present author, when he discovered it, felt much discouraged.

1897   *On A Form of Chronic Joint Disease in Children*

by George F. Still, M.A., M.D., M.R.C.P.

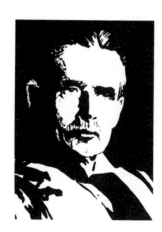

Medical Registrar and Pathologist to the Hospital for Sick Children Great Ormond St., London

The occasional occurrence in children of a disease closely resembling the rheumatoid arthritis of adults has been recognised for several years. The identity of the disease seen in children with that in adults has never, so far as I am aware, been called in question.

The purpose of the present paper is to show that although the disease known as rheumatoid arthritis in adults does undoubtedly occur in children, the disease which has most commonly been called rheumatoid arthritis in children differs both in its clinical aspect and in its morbid anatomy from the rheumatoid arthritis of adults; it presents, in fact, such marked differences as to suggest that it has a distinct pathology.

The cases hitherto grouped together as rheumatoid arthritis in children include, therefore, more than one disease; and it will be shown that there are at least three distinct joint affections which have thus been included under the one head, Rheumatoid arthritis.

The paper is based on a study of 22 cases, almost all of which have been in the Hospital for Sick Children, Great Ormond Street. Nineteen of these I have had under personal observation.

It will be necessary first to describe briefly the disease to which I have referred as the subject of this paper, and subsequently to point out the features of its clinical course and morbid anatomy, wherein it differs from the rheumatoid arthritis of adults.

The disease may be defined as a chronic progressive enlargement of joints, associated with general enlargement of glands and enlargement of spleen.

The onset is almost always before the second dentition; ten out of twelve cases began before the age of six years, and of these eight began within the first three years of life; the earliest was at fifteen months.

Girls are more commonly affected than boys; seven of the twelve cases were girls, five were boys.

The onset is usually insidious; the child, if old enough, complains of stiffness in one or more joints, which slowly become enlarged, and subsequently other joints become affected; but occasionally the onset is acute, with pyrexia and, it may be, with rigors.

I wish to lay some stress on the character of the enlargement of the joints. It feels and looks more like general thickening of the tissues round the joint than a bony enlargement, and is correspondingly smooth and fusiform, with none of the bony irregularity of the rheumatoid arthritis of adults.

The absence of osteophytic growth and of anything like bony lipping, even after years have elapsed since the outset, is striking.

There is, I believe, never any bony grating, although creaking, probably either of tendon or of cartilage, is frequently present. There is no redness or tenderness of the joints, except in very acute cases. The absence of pain is generally striking, but it may be present in slight degree, especially on movement. Limitation of movement, chiefly of extension, is almost always present; the child may be completely bedridden owing to more or less rigid flexion of joints.

The extensive deformities of the hands described by Charcot as occurring in the rheumatoid arthritis of adults (*Maladies des Vieillards*, 2nd ed., p. 201), are unknown to me in this disease. Those most common so far as I have seen are, flexion of the wrist with slight deviation of the hand to the ulnar side, and slight flexion of the proximal, combined sometimes with slight flexion of the distal, inter-phalangeal joint. Rarely there is slight hypertension of the metacarpo-phalangeal or proximal inter-phalangeal joint. The fingers may deviate very slightly to the radial side, but more often the deviation is at the proximal inter-phalangeal joint, and may be to either side; indeed, both directions may be seen in one hand. Adduction of the thumb was marked in one case.

The joints earliest affected were usually the knees, wrists and those of the cervical spine; the subsequent order of affection being ankles, elbows and fingers. The sterno-clavicular joint was affected in two out of twelve cases; the temporo-maxillary in three. The affection is symmetrical. There is no tendency to suppuration nor to bony ankylosis. The muscles which move the diseased joints show early and marked wasting, which contrasts often strongly with the good nutrition of the rest of the body.

The electrical reactions both to faradism and galvanism were brisk in three cases tested, but not otherwise altered.

Perhaps the most distinctive feature in these cases is the affection of the lymphatic glands. The enlargement is general, but affects primarily and chiefly those related to the joints affected. The glands are separate, rather hard than soft, not tender, and show no tendency to break down. They may become so large as to be visible. but more often do not become larger than a hazel-nut. The enlargement seems to bear a definite relation to the progress of the disease in the joints. Slight affection of the glands is found very soon after the first symptoms of the joint affection, and as the latter increases the glands become larger. If the joint affection subsides, the glands become smaller, increasing again in size if the joints become worse.

The glands most affected are the supra-trochlear, those along the brachial artery, and those in the axilla, also those in Scarpa's triangle, and deep in the iliac fossa along the iliac artery, and those in the posterior triangle of the neck. In one case I thought that the popliteal glands were enlarged, and in two cases there was some evidence clinically of enlarged mediastinal glands. I have never been able to make out enlargement of mesenteric glands, but in one of the autopsies which I shall mention, the glands in the hilum of the liver were found enlarged.

It will thus be seen that the enlargement is general; and I may add that it is constant; it was found in all the twelve cases mentioned.

Enlargement of the spleen is also a striking feature of these cases. It is, of course, not always easy to be certain of splenic enlargement, but it was definite and considerable in nine out of twelve cases, the edge of the spleen being felt one to two fingers' breadth below the costal margin. The enlargement of the spleen seems to be roughly proportionate to that of the glands, and like that of the glands has been observed to increase as the joint condition became worse.

The heart shows no evidence of valvular disease, but haemic bruits were detected in some of the cases.

There are some physical signs suggestive of adherent pericardium in two of the twelve cases, and in three other cases adherent pericardium was found quite unexpectedly at the autopsy.

Anaemia is generally present to some extent, but is seldom profound; the face has often a curious waxy pallor with flushed cheeks. The blood shows only moderate diminution of red corpuscles in most cases; in some, however, there is disproportionate deficiency of haemoglobin.

A curious symptom noticed in four cases out of the twelve, was slight prominence of the eyes, hardly enough to call exophthalmos, but enough to be noticeable. The thyroid seemed normal in the cases which I examined.

Sweating is often profuse, and not related to temperature. The temperature seems to be of two varieties: the one shows periods, generally lasting only a few days, of pyrexia followed by a longer interval of apyrexia; the other shows more or less continuous slight pyrexia. The pyrexial attacks occasionally show a curious regularity in their recurrence. One or two cases showed sudden attacks of hyperpyrexia, lasting one hour or two, and then subsiding rapidly. The pyrexial periods are not usually associated with any clinically

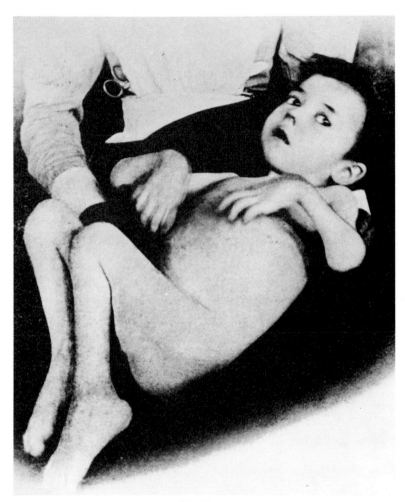

Still's Disease

demonstrable exacerbation of the joint trouble, nor indeed is it possible usually to find any definite cause for the fever.

A remarkable feature in these cases is the general arrest of development that occurs when the disease begins before the second dentition. A child of twelve and a half years would easily have been mistaken for six or seven years, while another of four years looked more like two and a half or three years.

The arrest is, however, of bodily rather than of mental development, and hence although backward in some respects from the enforced absence from school, the child often appears by comparison with its size to be rather precocious than backward.

The course of these cases is slow. Improvement may occur for a time under treatment or spontaneously, but the disease soon progresses again until a condition of general joint disease is reached which seems to be permanently stationary. The disease is not in itself fatal; the few deaths that have been recorded were due to complications.

Curiously enough, some accidental complications have been followed by marked improvement; thus I have known measles, scarlet fever, and catarrhal jaundice, to be each followed by distinct improvement of the joint symptoms.

The aetiology of the disease is very uncertain.

The morbid anatomy of this disease is gathered from three post-mortems. The joints show marked thickening of the capsule and of the connective tissue just outside this. There is also thickening and vascularisation, of the synovial membrane, and fibrous adhesions are sometimes present.

The cartilage may be perfectly normal, as in two cases that had lasted nearly one and a half years; but in a case that had lasted three years it showed pitting of its surface as if from pressure, with little processes of the thickened synovial membrane fitting accurately into the pits, which were situated chiefly at the margin of the cartilage; otherwise, however, the cartilage was healthy—there was no fibrillation, no osteophytic change, no exposure or eburnation of bone.

The enlarged glands appear normal on section, or show small ecchymoses in their substance.

The spleen weighed in each case about 5 ounces, so that it was considerably enlarged; it was firm, and appeared normal on section.

In each case the pericardium was universally adherent; there were also pleural adhesions. There was no endocarditis certainly in two cases, but in the third the mitral valve was perhaps a little thickened.

In conclusion, I should like just to mention another affection which I have known raise the question of rheumatoid arthritis in a child. It is a rare form of syphilitic joint disease. It shows, in addition to the commoner chronic effusion with thickening of capsule in medium-sized and larger joints, definite bony thickening and lipping, which affects also the smaller joints; this osteophytic change may even simulate Herberden's nodes, as I have seen in a boy six years old, in whom some of the distal phalanges showed lateral thickenings very like Heberden's nodes. They were, however, less regular in their distribution, for they occurred not only on the distal, but also on one or two of the proximal phalangeal joints, and the toes showed similar nodosities. In this boy the larger joints showed chronic effusion, with some thickening of surrounding soft tissues, and there was a gumma over one ulna, and further evidence of syphilis was found in old iritis. There was no enlargement of glands or spleen.

It may be useful to sum up the conclusions arrived at in this paper.

There is a disease, occurring in children, and beginning before the second dentition, which is characterised clinically by elastic fusiform enlargement of joints without bony change, and also by enlargement of glands and spleen.

This disease has hitherto been called rheumatoid arthritis, but it differs from the disease in adults, clinically in the absence of bony change, even when the disease is advanced, and in the enlargement of glands and spleen, and pathologically in the absence, even in an advanced case, of the cartilage changes which are found quite early in that disease, and also in the absence of osteophytic change.

These differences are not to be attributed merely to modification of disease by difference of age, as there occurs also in children a disease in every respect identical with the rheumatoid arthritis of adults.

Under the head of Rheumatoid Arthritis in children, at least three conditions have been confused which are both clinically and pathologically distinct, namely:- (1) the joint disease described in the present paper; (2) a disease identical with the rheumatoid arthritis of adults; (3) a disease probably identical with that described by Jaccoud as chronic fibrous rheumatism.

Charcot's Joints: Jean-Martin Charcot, 1825-1893

Charcot was the son of a Parisian coach-builder of limited means. Legend has it that Father sent his three sons to school for a year. The son who did best could have higher education, the middle son would be trained for the army, and the son who came bottom would follow his father's footsteps as a coach-builder.

Jean-Martin came top and graduated in medicine. While working as an interne at the Salpêtrière, he wrote a thesis in which he distinguished between gout and rheumatoid arthritis for the first time. He spent the rest of his life at the Salpêtrière, becoming, in 1882, the first Professor of nervous diseases in the world. He was world famous in his own day largely because of the splendid demonstrations and lectures that he devised. He was one of the first to break away from the tradition of bedside teaching. He gave a lecture in a hall, well lighted and equipped with a magic lantern and brought the patients to illustrate points in his lecture, which he demonstrated in a most theatrical manner; and he started the fashion, which is so well kept up by neurologists today, of imitating any neurological disturbance from a minor nerve palsy to grand mal epilepsy.

He wrote a great deal; in his lectures and papers can be found first descriptions of intermittent claudication, disseminated sclerosis, amyotrophic lateral sclerosis, intermittent hepatic fever, neuropathic joint disease, and oddities such as herpes zoster due to compression of the posterior root ganglion.

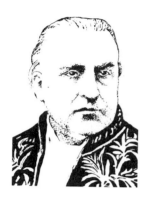

Charcot's Joints: 1868

I desire, at present, to insist upon an affection, whose existence I have pointed out, and which I am accustomed to designate, in order to prejudge nothing, by the name of *arthropathy of ataxic patients*.

To my mind, and I hope to make you share my way of looking at it, we have here one of the manifold forms of spinal arthropathy. What is spinal arthropathy, some amongst you may ask? I have proposed to designate by this name a whole group of articular affections, which appear to depend directly on certain lesions of the spinal cord, with which, consequently, they should be connected as symptomatic affections. The irritative lesions of the spinal cord, especially those which occupy the grey substance, react sometimes, you are aware, on the periphery, and determine various nutritive disorders, either in the skin or in the deeper parts, such as the muscles. The bones and articulations do not appear to escape this law. It follows that the arthropathies of locomotor ataxia would be, according to my judgement, one of the forms of these articular affections, developed under the more or less direct influence of lesion of the spinal centre.

Here, it may not be useless to make you remark that all the articular affections which supervene, in a patient attacked with locomotor ataxia, do not necessarily come within the following description. Thus, it is not rare to see nodose rheumatism, common dry arthritis, coincide with ataxia. Then, and on this point I would insist, these rheumatic affections show themselves with their accustomed symptoms. Ataxic arthropathy, on the contrary, is evolved with clinical characteristics, altogether its own, as you will soon see, which cause it to constitute a really distinct disorder.

I would also add that there is no question here of an extremely rare and exceptional phenomenon. I can show you five examples of these arthropathies in about fifty ataxic patients, whom I know in this refuge. Five cases in fifty, is already a respectable number. Taking my own experience, I have observed this complication of ataxia, perhaps thirty times, in private practice and in hospital.

A woman aged 49 was admitted to the Salpêtrière on May 1, 1867. She had begun to suffer from symptoms of locomotor ataxy ten years previously, and she had been bedridden for the past four years. She noticed on awakening in the morning of June 9, 1860, that her left shoulder was swollen, the swelling getting progressively less until it reached the wrist. She was not feverish, there was no pain, and she was quite unable to account for the swelling.

Three days later the swelling had disappeared from the arm and the forearm, but the shoulder still remained larger than normal, and there was marked creaking when the joint moved.

On June 18, in addition to the general swelling of the shoulder, there was a rounded swelling about the size of an orange situated in front of the joint. It fluctuated, and appeared to be a distended subdeltoid bursa. The creaking in the joint was still more marked. Matters remained in this state until August 2, when the patient was seized with diarrhoea, choleraic in character, of which she died on August 15. The swollen shoulder became much smaller a few days before death.

A post-mortem examination made on August 16 showed that the capsule of the joint was much thickened, and contained some bony plates in its substance. The synovial membrane was also thickened, and was slightly reddened on its inner surface. The cavity of the joint contained a little transparent yellow fluid, and there were intra-articular loose bodies. The head of the humerus had undergone the

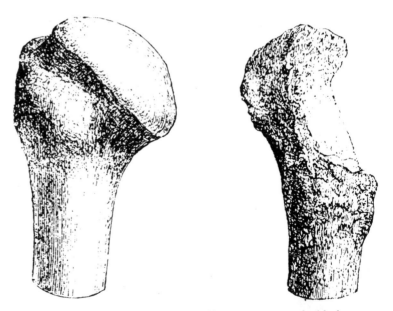

Charcot's Joints: A normal head of humerus compared with that of the patient.

remarkable changes shown in the accompanying figure. Although the arthropathy had only lasted nine weeks, a large part of the head of the bone had disappeared as if it had been rubbed away by friction. There was no trace of the articular cartilage, and the globular head was replaced by a flat or slightly concave surface, worn away and roughened in some parts, smooth and eburnated in others. A few small rounded osteophytes surrounded this surface, but they were quite unlike the bony edges which surround and enlarge the joint surfaces in osteo-arthritis.

The glenoid cavity showed similar changes. The surface was worn away like the head of the humerus, but to a lesser extent. Every trace of articular cartilage had disappeared, and there was no lipping of the bone. The clavicle and acromion were normal in appearance. The posterior columns of the spinal cord showed in a high degree the lesions of grey degeneration with atrophy, more especially in the dorsal and lumbar regions. The cervical cord was affected in the same way, but to a less extent. The posterior nerve-roots were clearly atrophied and of a greyish colour. There were slight traces of a posterior spinal meningitis.

I shall confine myself, gentlemen, to this summary exposition, which suffices, indeed, to make you familiar with the principal aspects of the arthropathy.

A. To sum up: without appreciable external cause, without blow or fall, apart from any traumatic accident whatever, the local affection appears. At this moment the inco-ordination is not yet marked, the patients do not *fling* about their legs, in a disorderly manner. I must insist on this detail, because it answers an objection made by Herr Volkmann, which has been repeated by other surgeons, who refuse to see, in the arthropathy of ataxic patients, anything else than a traumatic arthritis caused by the mode of locomotion peculiar to these patients.

Nor can you invoke here, either the influence of cold, or a diathetic state, gout, rheumatism, &c., to account for it; the articular affections due to these causes, have, moreover, a totally different physiognomy.

B. This arthropathy is developed at a *but slightly advanced period of the spinal disease*, and most commonly when its symptomatology is limited to the lightning pains. The inco-ordination, it is true, does not generally make its appearance when the arthropathy has occurred. Thus it has, as you observe, its place marked for it in the regular succession of the symptoms of locomotor ataxia.

C. The arthropathy is produced, generally, without prodromes, if we except, however, those *cracking sounds* which we find mentioned in a certain number of cases.

E. Most usually, the first phenomenon discernible is extreme tumefaction of the entire member, no previous difficulty in its movements having existed. This tumefaction is formed—1°, by a considerable hydrarthrosis; 2°, by an engorgement which, in the majority of cases, presents a hard consistence, and in which the ordinary symptoms of oedema are not generally very marked.

This arthropathy is not commonly accompanied by fever, or by pains; these symptoms are only exceptionally recorded on the notes.

At the end of some weeks, or of some months, the swelling disappears and then all returns to the normal state (*benignant form*); sometimes, on the contrary, serious disorders remain in the joints, crackings, dislocations, answering to a wearing down of the osseous surfaces, and various luxations (*malignant form*). In spite of these profound lesions, the member affected by arthropathy may still serve for prehension, if it be the upper extremity; or for walking, if the hip and knee be the articulation affected. Naturally, this partial freedom of motion diminishes if the inco-ordination makes progress, or the luxation becomes exaggerated.

F. With respect to the question of frequency, the order of preference begins with the knee, then comes the shoulder, next the elbow, the hips, and the wrists. But the small articulations are not always spared.

It is proper now, gentlemen, to examine what information is supplied us by pathological anatomy. Undoubtedly, in cases of old standing, when the articular surfaces, worn and deprived of cartilage, have continued to move on each other, the limbs being still made use of more or less imperfectly, the signs observed are those of dry arthritis; to wit, eburnation and deformation of the articular surfaces, deformation of the osseous extremities, bony burrs and stalactites, foreign bodies, &c.

There are, however, two points to which I must request your attention.

1°. The predominance of wearing away over the production of bony burrs in recent cases. Compare, for instance, the humerus which I show you and which comes from an ataxic patient, who succumbed two months after the commencement of the arthropathy, with the plate of Adams's work, representing the lesions of scapulo-humeral dry arthritis, and you will comprehend what reasons I have for insisting on this.

2°. I shall mention, in the second place, the frequency of true luxations, which are, to some extent, the rule in ataxic arthropathy, when the articulations admit such displacement—in the shoulder, for instance—while they are only exceptions in common dry arthritis, in which they are usually apparent, and not real.

A. Again, we are today well acquainted with the articular affections which result from lesions of the peripheral nerves in the same way as herpes, glossy skin, rapid muscular atrophy, and so many other trophic disorders of the same kind. The observations relating to wounds received in battle, which were noted by Dr. Weir Mitchell, during the American War, and published anew in a recent work, are very instructive, in this respect.

B. You are acquainted, likewise, with those singular articular affections which become developed in limbs smitten with hemi-plegia, owing to haemorrhage or ramollissement of the brain, at a certain period of the disease, and which come anatomically under the description of acute or sub-acute arthritis.

C. But, to speak only of what specially concerns the spinal cord, I believe I can declare that there is, perhaps, not one of the morbid forms to which it is subject which may not provoke, in certain circumstances, an articular affection manifestly correlated as a symptom of the lesion of this department of the nervous centres.

We observe these arthropathies especially:—1°, in paraplegia from Pott's disease: 2°, in acute myelitis; 3°, in certain cases of tumours primarily occupying the spinal grey substance (Gull); 4°, in certain cases of lesions of the grey substance determining progressive muscular atrophy (Rosenthal, Remak, Patruban); 5°, but the case in which it is most easy to demonstrate the connection which exists, according to my opinion, between the spinal lesion and the articular affection is that of traumatic lesions affecting the spinal cord.

We should now pause to seek what may be the mechanism which presides over the development of these arthropathies, and what, in particular, is the region of the spinal cord the alteration of which determines the articular lesion; for, manifestly, all the regions of the spinal centre cannot be indiscriminately arraigned. Reverting to locomotor ataxia, where this question has been especially studied, it is clear that, *a priori*, the arthropathy could not be referred to the common and trite lesion of the posterior columns. We must look elsewhere.

Notwithstanding the desideratum which I have noticed above, I would recommend gentlemen, to your close attention, the arthropathy of ataxia as a pathological and clinical fact of genuine worth. As regards the first point, we have here an element for the solution of an interesting problem of pathological physiology. Clinically, you will learn to know an affection which, if you take up the right point of view, may contribute to elucidate the diagnosis and to avoid deplorable errors. How often have not I seen persons, not yet familiar with this arthropathy, misunderstand its real nature, and, wholly preoccupied with the local affection, even absolutely forget that behind the disease of the joint there was a disease far more important in character, and which in reality dominated the situation —sclerosis of the posterior columns.

4 NEUROMUSCULAR DISEASE

Cerebral Palsy: William John Little, 1810-1894

Little's life was largely shaped by the fact that he had polio as a child, resulting in a left talipes equino varus deformity. He went to school in France, and after working for an apothecary for a while, studied at the London Hospital.

Two years after qualifying he went to the Continent ostensibly to study. He had tried all sorts of mechanical contraptions to correct his deformity without success, and heard that Stromeyer was pioneering tenotomy for the condition in Hanover. Everyone told him it was dreadful and valueless, but after watching Stromeyer at work for some time, he decided that it was the treatment for him. He had an Achilles tenotomy and his deformity was much improved. He helped in Stromeyer's clinic for a while and then started to tenotomise in Germany. He wrote a thesis for an M.D. on this, and returned to England to introduce the operation here. He persuaded his friends to subscribe to a hospital for him. This became the Royal Orthopaedic Hospital which was amalgamated to form the Royal National Orthopaedic Hospital in London.

He had wanted to become a surgeon but was deterred when he missed a post at the London Hospital that he had coveted. Instead he decided to become a physician and after a period as Assistant Physician was elected to the staff of the London Hospital at the age of 35.

He wrote on all aspects of club foot. He advocated tenotomy of any tendon producing deformity whereas Stromeyer had only divided the tendon Achilles; Stromeyer called him the "Apostle of Tenotomy". He also wrote on other deformities such as knock knee and scoliosis, described the spastic state arising from birth damage of the brain known as Little's disease, and pioneered the use of intravenous saline and alcohol for dehydration.

At the age of 53 his private practice kept him too busy to go to the London Hospital, and he retired from there, but kept his practice going for another twenty years.

It is interesting that his paper on cerebral palsy was read before the Obstetrical Society.

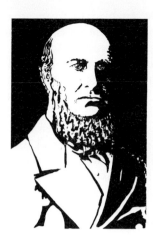

Little's Disease: 1862

ON THE INFLUENCE OF ABNORMAL PARTURITION, DIFFICULT LABOURS, PREMATURE BIRTH, AND ASPHYXIA NEONATORUM, ON THE MENTAL AND PHYSICAL CONDITION OF THE CHILD, ESPECIALLY IN RELATION TO DEFORMITIES

by W. J. Little, M.D.

Senior Physician to the London Hospital; founder of the Royal Orthopaedic Hospital; Visiting-Physician to Asylum for Idiots, Earslwood; etc.

Pathology has gradually taught that the foetus in utero is subject to similar diseases to those which afflict the economy at later periods of existence. This is especially true if we turn to the study of the special class of abnormal conditions, which are termed deformities.

There is, however, an epoch of existence, viz., the period of birth, during which, at first sight, we might consider that the foetal organism is subjected to conditions so different to those of its earlier and of its prospective later existence, that any untoward influences applied at this important juncture would affect the economy in a manner different to the influences at work during the periods ordinarily characterised as those of before birth and after birth.

The object of this communication is to show that the act of birth does occasionally imprint upon the nervous and muscular systems of the nascent infantile organism very serious and peculiar evils. When we investigate the evils in question, and their causative influences, we find that the same laws of pathology apply to diseases incidental to the act of birth as to those which originate before and after birth. We are, in fact, afforded another illustration that there exists no such thing as exceptional or special pathology.

Nearly twenty years ago, in a course of lectures published in the *Lancet*, and more fully in a *Treatise on Deformities*, published in 1853, I showed that premature birth, difficult labours, mechanical injuries during parturition to head and neck, where life had been saved, convulsions following the act of birth, were apt to be succeeded by a determinate affection of the limbs of the child, which I designated spastic rigidity of the limbs of new-born children, spastic rigidity from asphyxia neonatorum, and assimilated it to the trismus nascentium and the universal spastic rigidity sometimes produced at later periods of existence.

It is obvious that the great majority of apparently stillborn infants, whose lives are saved by the attendant accoucheur, recover unharmed from that condition. I have, however, witnessed so many cases of deformity, mental and physical, traceable to causes operative at birth, that I consider the subject worthy the notice of the Obstetrical Society. In orthopaedic practice alone, during about twenty years, I have met with probably two hundred cases of spastic rigidity from this cause. I omit reckoning the subjects of idiot and other asylums, in which probably such cases abound, but of which I have been able to attain no history. I revert to the subject at the present moment because I believe I am now enabled to form an opinion of the nature of the anatomical lesions and the particular abnormal event at birth on which the symptoms depend. Moreover, as the study of the proximate cause of the affections which I shall describe requires the light of such facts as the members of this society have peculiar opportunities of supplying, I make no further apology for occupying the Society's time.

Before I describe the mental and physical derangements of the infant which can be referred to the effects of abnormal parturition and asphyxia at birth, I may be permitted to dwell upon the principal phenomena which occur in the foetal organism immediately before, during, and immediately after, the act of normal parturition.

The detailed autopsies of Hecker and Weber, with the carefully appended histories of the nature of the fatal impediment at birth, have greatly facilitated an explanation of the spastic rigidity and paralysis of limbs, which appeared from my observations to be produced by so many different forms of unnatural parturition. The dissections of these obstetricians show the important fact that mechanical injury of the foetal head, neck, or trunk, is not necessary for the production of intense congestion and blood extravasation of serous surfaces of chest, brain and spinal cord. The other phenomenon commonly observed in difficult and abnormal parturition is that of interruption of placental respiration and circulation with non-substitution of pulmonary breathing and circulation. To this phenomenon alone, when mechanical injury or impediment has not existed, can we attribute the internal congestions, capillary extravasations, serous effusions which correspond with, or produce the symptoms of asphyxia, suspended animation, apoplexy, torpidity, tetanic spasms, convulsions of new-born children, and the spastic rigidity, paralysis, and idiocy subsequently witnessed. I am justified in regarding the dissections of Hecker and Weber as confirmatory of the opinion emitted by me, that asphyxia neonatorum, through resulting injury to nervous centres, is the cause of the commonest contractions which originate at the moment of birth, namely, more or less general spastic rigidity, and sometimes of paralytic contraction.

The former class of affections may be described as impairment of volition, with tonic rigidity and ultimately structural shortening, in varying degrees, of a few or many of the muscles of the body. Both lower extremities are more or less generally involved. Sometimes the affection of one limb only is observed by the parent, but examination usually shows a smaller degree of affection in the limb supposed to be sound. The contraction in the hips, knees, and ankles, is often considerable. The flexors and adductors of thighs, the flexors of knees, and the gastrocnemii, preponderate. In most cases, after a time, owing to structural shortening of the muscles and of the articular ligaments, and perhaps to some change of form of articular surfaces, the thighs cannot be completely abducted or extended, the knees cannot be straightened, nor can the heels be properly applied to the ground. The upper extremities are sometimes held down by preponderating action of pectorals, teres major and teres minor, and latissimus dorsi; the elbows are semi-flexed, the wrists partially flexed, pronated, and the fingers incapable of perfect voluntary direction. Sometimes the upper extremities appear unaffected with spasm or want of volition, sometimes a mere awkwardness in using them exists. Not unfrequently the parent reports that the hands were formerly affected. Participation of the muscles of trunk is sometimes shown by the shortened, flattened aspect of pectoral and abdominal surfaces, as compared with the more elongated and rounded form of the back. The prominence of back partially disappears on recumbency, but the greater weakness of muscles on dorsal aspect of trunk is obvious when the individual again attempts to sit upright. The muscles feel harder than natural to the age. Micturition is sometimes observed to be rare, and the bowels usually confined, either from deficient exercise of voluntary expulsive power or from implication of the sphincters. The muscles of speech are commonly involved, varying in degree from inability to utter correctly particular letters up to entire loss of articulating power. Sometimes articulation is only slow and difficult, like other acts of volition, the child or adult reminding us of a tardigrade animal. Sometimes the speech is nervous, impulsive or stuttering. Often during the earliest months of life deglutition is impaired, and the power of carrying saliva into the fauces is not acquired until late. The intellectual functions are sometimes quite unaffected, but in the majority of cases the intellect suffers—from the slightest impairment which the parent unwillingly acknowledges or fails to perceive, up to entire imbecility. The functions of organic life are unexceptionally performed, except, perhaps, that of development of caloric, although the depression of the temperature in later life is more properly dependent upon the want of proper exercise. The frame is often lean and wiry, but not wasted. On the contrary, it is generally well nourished. The appetite is good, the child is often described as the healthiest of the family. These subjects often lead a more precarious existence during the first weeks after birth, at first even vegetative existence langishes, sometimes, perhaps, because premature birth or difficult labour, by impairing the maternal supply of nutriment, renders more difficult the infant's recovery from the shock its system received at birth. However, in the majority of instances, after restoration of the vegetative functions, a gradual but slow amelioration of all the functions of animal life is perceived. Some cases present distinct convulsive twitchings of face or limbs during first days after birth, open or suppressed convulsions, opisthotonos, or laryngismus. In some instances the persistent rigidity of muscles commences or is observed shortly after birth, in others it escapes observation until the lapse of some weeks or months. The child's limbs are sometimes reported to have been simply weaker, to have shared in the general debility, the question of viability having alone occupied the attention of the attendants during the first month. Occasionally the weakness of the limbs has been recognised as a genuine paralysis in the first instance, of which the rigidity of the muscles has been the sequel. Before the age of three or four months, though sometimes in slight cases not until ordinary time for walking arrives, the nurse perceives that the infant never thoroughly straightens the knees, that these cannot be properly depressed or separated, that she is unable to wash and dress the infant with the ordinary facility, that the hands are not properly used. The upper extremities recover before the lower limbs. Sometimes the trunk is habitually stiffened, so that the infant is turned over in the lap "all of a piece", as the nurse expresses it. Occasionally the head is habitually retracted. Where the symptom of convulsions or "inward convulsions" exists, the rigidity is attributed to the convulsions. In many cases convulsions have been absent. As the child approaches the period at which the first attempts at standing and progression should be made, it is observed to make no use of the limbs, or he is incapable of standing except on the toes, or the feet are disposed to cross each other. Even children slightly affected rarely "go alone" before three or four years of age, many are unable to raise themselves from the ground at that age, and others do not walk, even indifferently, at puberty. On examination, the surgeon finds that the soles of the feet are not properly applied to the ground, that the knees always incline inwardly, and continue bent. When locomotion is accomplished, the movements are characterised by inability to stand still and balance the body in erect attitude. In the best recoveries from *general* spastic rigidity, even in the adult, the gait is shuffling, stiff; each knee, by forcible spastic rubbing against its fellow, obstructs progression.

The external form of cranium occasionally exhibits departure from the normal or average type, such as general smallness of skull, depression of frontal or occipital region only, sometimes one lateral half of skull, sometimes of one half of occiput, or forehead only. In slight cases the head has been well developed.

In cases even with great inertia as to exercise of volition in any part of the body, common sensibility appears little, if at all, deficient. The child often, indeed, manifests uncommon sensitiveness to external impressions, even when approaching adolescence he is alarmed at trifling noises. The sleep after the first weeks of life is light, easily disturbed. Often there is extreme sensibility to touch, the whole condition reminding the observer of tetanus. In a few cases a distinct resemblance to severe chorea is perceptible.

Brachial Plexus Injuries

The obstetricians are said to have been the first to observe these injuries, though I have been unable to locate Smellie's account amongst the hundreds of case reports that he published.

Duchenne of Boulogne introduced the subject of obstetrical palsies in 1855 and 22 years later Erb began to locate the site of the lesion by studying the pattern of paralysis. Klumpke then distinguished the different varieties of paralysis that could occur bringing animal experiments to support her ideas of the mechanism of some of the features.

It is interesting that of the five cases Erb marshalls to support his argument that brachial plexus paralyses often conform to a pattern, only one of the cases would today be called an Erb's palsy. Two of his patients appear to have had cervical spondylosis, one was a Pancoast syndrome, another is not clearly one thing or another, only his last case—included almost as an afterthought—is an Erb's Palsy. It is remarkable that on the basis of these miscellaneous cases he should have accurately localised the site of a group of brachial plexus injuries, which every medical student knows as Erb's point.

I guess that Erb wrote this paper after reading the challenge that Duchenne threw out 22 years before when he described this birth injury. It explains Erb's rather obtuse title.

Duchenne described four cases of upper trunk birth palsies.

> "In this kind of paralysis of the upper limb from obstetrical manipulations, the arm falls motionless along the side of the body, and is rotated inwards; the forearm remains extended, but the movements of the hand are preserved.
>
> "I leave to others the study of the anatomical cause, and to say why in these cases the same muscles (deltoid, infraspinatus, biceps and brachialis) are always paralysed".

Wilhelm Heinrich Erb, 1840-1921

"Erb's fame was made possible by hard work over a long period of time, with close attention to detail."

The son of a woodsman in the Black Forest, Erb studied at Heidelburg. His interest in clinical neurology developed when he worked for Friedreich. Erb was a prolific writer; on returning from his holidays, he usually produced a new piece of work. In all he wrote 237 papers and several books, one of peripheral nerve diseases, a textbook of spinal cord diseases, and another on electrotherapy. In 1880 he succeeded Friedreich at Heidelburg. He founded a journal, and was first President of the Society of German Neurologists in 1907.

Erb did much to give clinical examination of the nervous system its present form. He pointed out the significance and value of pupillary and tendon reflexes. He is remembered for his account of brachial plexus injuries.

In manner he was brusque and intense, and offended people by language unusual in academic circles; he was more respected than loved. Medical administration, education and local politics were subsidiary interests. He died, it is said, whilst listening to his favourite symphony, the Beethoven Eroica.

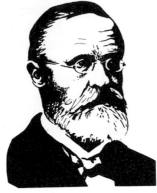

Concerning an Unusual Localisation of Brachial Plexus Paralyses

W. Erb, 1877

When reviewing the case histories of my material with reference to peripheral paralyses of the upper extremity there was remarkable uniformity of the muscles affected by the paralysis. The paralysis was not exclusively localised to one of the main branches of the brachial plexus but to lesser branches with the exception of the ulnar nerve. The paralyses of the various branches of the brachial plexus are sufficiently known and their effects have been sufficiently studied; however this is not true of paralyses of the individual roots which form the brachial plexus (the anterior branches of the cervical nerves).

It would be desirable to understand the localisation and effects of the various syndromes that can occur. It must be assumed that each root is always composed of the same motor and sensory fibres; then one is in a position to determine the site of the lesion in one or other of the roots on the basis of the motor and sensory deficit.

He describes 4 cases to demonstrate this.

Case 1. Konrad Sauer, 52 years old, a ropemaker. The condition had been present for 5 weeks after carrying a heavy load on his head. It began with pain and stiffness on the left side of the neck and of the left shoulder radiating down the arm to the fingers. At the same time a feeling of numbness affected the thumb and index fingers; there was such a degree of weakness of the arm that the patient could no longer lift it. On examination there was complete paralysis of the left deltoid, biceps, brachialis, and brachioradialis. The supinator also appeared much weakened. The remaining shoulder muscles, triceps, all the forearm muscles and all the small muscles of the hand were normal.

The sense of touch of the thumb and index finger was slightly reduced. Electrical examination revealed an incomplete reaction of degeneration. The muscles were slightly tender on palpation and atrophied during the course of the disease.

Treatment: The patient was treated by galvanism, and was discharged cured after 7 weeks. This case was evidently a traumatic neuritis of a part of the brachial plexus.

His second case developed after a fall in which the shoulder received a little of the impact. The neurological deficit was the same as the first case. 'Satisfactory' improvement occurred after six months.

The third case was of spontaneous onset.

The fourth case presented with the same neurological deficit and hard supraclavicular glands. He died soon afterwards from carcinomatosis.

54

The fact that these four cases had a similar neurological deficit led him to suggest that the lesion was at the same place in them all.

> It is probable that the lesion in the cases mentioned was localised to the fifth or sixth cervical roots or their anterior branches or at the junction of them both.

He recalls that similar cases are found in the new-born, due to birth injury, and were first described by Duchenne. Biceps, brachialis, deltoid and sometimes infraspinatus are paralysed. Secondary contractures develop giving rise to a very characteristic deformity of the arm.

> I have myself observed a case in an infant which had been delivered two months before after a version and subsequent extraction. I found the arm rather mobile, flaccid, and lay extended by the side of the trunk, in a position of full internal rotation, the wrist and fingers were flexed and moved little. More precise observation, which is so difficult in infants, showed complete paralysis of the deltoid, biceps, brachialis, and possibly of brachio-radialis and infraspinatus. There was marked weakness of all the muscles innervated by the radial nerve. Finally there was a secondary contracture of the pectoralis major.

He thought that it was most likely that the plexus was compressed during this difficult delivery. The lesion must be high up in the neck in the region of the scalene muscles. He considered the paralysis of the infraspinatus an important clue to the localisation of the lesion and one which should be carefully looked for in the future.

Madame Auguste Déjerine-Klumpke, 1859-1927

Auguste Klumpke was one of the first woman doctors in Paris and described whilst a student the brachial palsy that bears her name. She must have eased the way for women who wished to follow her.

She was born in San Francisco, educated in Lausanne, and, with her four sisters, arrived in Paris at the age of 18 determined to overcome the hostility which women who wished to study medicine met at this time. Her sisters all achieved distinction; one as a musician, another as an artist and the third became a Doctor of Science.

In her final year as a student she married Jules Déjerine, who later achieved fame as a neurologist at the Salpêtrière. Auguste helped him with his study of neuroanatomy and when he died in 1917 founded an institute to commemorate him and allow his work to go on.

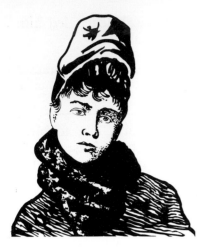

Klumpke's Paralysis: 1885

Contribution to the Study of Radicular Paralyses of the Brachial Plexus

The paralysis of the upper roots, generally known as Erb's palsy, is certainly the best studied and most widely recognised of all the radicular paralyses of the brachial plexus.

At other times, however, one has to deal with a total paralysis of the upper limb in which the group of muscles affected in the Duchenne-Erb paralysis recover leaving the whole of the lower part of the arm paralysed: this is a paralysis of the lower roots of the brachial plexus.

Then what constitutes this complete brachial plexus paralysis, which can remain the same or at a given moment can change into the upper type or become lower type? Like the upper palsy, it is produced by violent injury—a fall, after a blow on the shoulder, after a gunshot wound, or following reduction of a dislocated shoulder.

Here the palsy affects the hand and forearm as well as the shoulder; it is flail; but while the sensory loss is slight or missing in the upper type, it is practically never absent in the combined or lower varieties. The anaesthesia is complete for the forearm and hand. In the majority of cases it extends for one or two finger-breadths above the elbow, limited there by a more or less irregular boundary. Occasionally it extends over the arm, but it is always the outer and posterior aspect up to the level of the deltoid insertion that are affected by this sensory disturbance. The skin of the inner aspect of the arm and that of the shoulder always remains unaffected, since the lesion is definitely limited to the brachial plexus. The sparing of the inner aspect of the arm is easily explained since it is innervated by the intercosto-brachial nerve and branches of the medial cutaneous nerve of the arm; the former takes its origin from perforating branches of the second and third intercostals and the latter receives anastomotic branches from the same source.

Depending on the severity of the injury, the motor and sensory disturbances may be slight or may, on the other hand, be accompanied by the complications of serious injuries of the peripheral nerves: muscular atrophy, loss of electrical reactions, trophic changes, glossy skin, loss of sweating, cyanosis, increase or reduction of skin temperature, subcutaneous adiposity, fibrous ankylosis, etc., etc.

There is another sign mentioned in all communications, a sign pathognomonic of lower root paralysis, a sign that is not found in complete plexus palsies which are to become the Duchenne-Erb variety: this is the oculo-pupillary phenomenon.

This sign, which is constant in all true lower root palsies, is characterised by myosis, narrowing of the palpebral fissure, and in some cases by the eyeball retracting and becoming smaller. Furthermore in three cases one has noticed flattening of the cheek on the side corresponding with the paralysis.

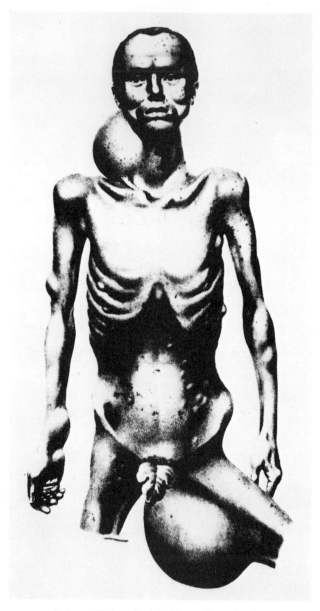

Robert William Smith: Neurofibromatosis

Neurofibromatosis: Robert William Smith, 1807-1873

Robert Smith was born in Dublin, studied and worked there, at a time when Irish medicine was very active: Stokes, Corrigan, Colles, Graves and Adams set the pace. Smith was a surgical pathologist at heart—a great collector of specimens of bone pathology, especially fractures.

He founded the Pathological Society at Dublin and when Colles died in 1843, Smith, at Colles' request, performed the autopsy, a report of which was published.

He had a small surgical practice and in 1847 wrote a very thoughtful book on fractures. In this he mentions the supination injury of wrist which is known after him, and a description of Madelung's deformity before Madelung described it. In 1849 he published a work on neuromata, which is said to be the largest book published in Ireland up to that time. When it is opened it is larger than an ordinary dining-room table. Smith wrote on neurofibromatosis very fully before von Recklinghausen described it in 1882, and for this reason his account is included.

He became Professor of Surgery at Trinity College, Dublin, and gave up his practice to teach.

A Treatise on the Pathology, Diagnosis, and Treatment of Neuroma

by Robert William Smith, 1849

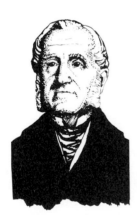

Although numerous instances of solitary neuroma have been placed on record, the annals of pathology contain as yet but few examples in which neuromatous tumours have been developed in almost countless numbers throughout the greater part of the nervous system: not only connected with the deep seated trunks, but visible in almost every superficial nerve of the body; not limited to the extremities, but likewise involving the nerves of the great cavities; not confined to the cerebro-spinal, but also implicating the grand sympathetic system; not the seat of pain, but on the contrary, the source of no apparent injury to the patient; unaccompanied by any lesion of innervation, even when such nerves as the vagus and phrenic are involved from one extremity to the other.

John McCann, 35 years of age, was admitted into the Richmond Hospital, under the care of Dr. Hutton in 1840, having a large tumour on the right side of the neck, of a globular form, and equal to a moderate-sized coconut in magnitude; it extended from within the mastoid process to within a short distance of the sterno-clavicular articulation. It presented a uniform surface, and admitted of being moved freely in a transverse direction, but could neither be pushed upwards nor drawn downwards; the external jugular vein grooved its surface, the integuments did not adhere to it (nor although it obviously extended deep into the neck) did it appear to have contracted a close adhesion to any important part. It was solid throughout and had existed for upwards of fifteen years, but it had never been painful nor was it now the source of much inconvenience to the patient.

A second tumour, about as large as a walnut, existed underneath the left side of the tongue. (*Treatment was decided against.*)

In 1843 he was again taken into hospital, having on the day previous . . . been found . . . lying upon the side of the road complaining of a pain in the left hip. A large solid tumour was discovered upon the back of the thigh, which the man stated had been growing for nearly two years. It exceeded in magnitude the size of the head of the patient. Its general surface was smooth. Several large veins ramified beneath the integuments, which were not adherent to the tumour. The patient suffered no acute pain. His general health had undergone a material alteration since the period of his first admission into hospital; he was now pale and greatly emaciated. . . .

Upon the day succeeding that upon which the patient died I made a careful examination of the body. . . . The largest (tumour) was situated upon the posterior part of the right thigh, immediately beneath the lower margin of the gluteus maximus muscle; it was of an oblong form and considerably larger than a lemon. There was one upon the outer side of the right arm, near its centre, of the size of a pigeon's egg; and another upon the front of the right forearm, immediately above the carpus, nearly as large as a hen's egg: they all admitted being moved in a lateral direction. The intercostal spaces upon each side, as well as the abdominal parietes and the right inguinal region, presented numerous tumours about the size of large peas.

He then goes on to describe the detailed autopsy findings; he found 150 tumours on the right lumbar plexus and its branches, and similar numbers on the sciatic and brachial plexuses. One tumour on the sciatic nerve measured 11 in. by 10 in.

In this remarkable case the total number of tumours exceeded 800; they presented a striking uniformity, both in their external characters and the internal structure; their form was oval or oblong; their colour, a yellowish white; they were solid, and each surrounded by a capsule, which was continuous with the neurilemma; their surface was smooth; their long axis corresponded with the direction of the nerve on which they exist, and they were only movable from side to side. Their section exhibited an exceedingly dense, close texture, of a whitish colour, and a somewhat glistening aspect, presenting a uniform degree of solidarity, and remarkable for a total absence of vascularity. Examined by the aid of a microscope, they were found to be composed essentially of a fibro-cellular structure, the fibrous tissue predominating in by far the greatest number, the areolar predominating in a few; the fibres arranged in bands or loops, amongst which permanent oval or elongated nuclei became apparent on the addition of acetic acid. In no one instance was there any trace discovered of nerve tubes, nor any indication of malignant disease.

Sciatica

The best early description of sciatica comes from a monograph by Cotugno written in 1764. About 90 years later pathologists found necropsy evidence of disc protusion. Another 90 years passed before it was realised that there was any connection between these two observations.

Virchow gave a brief account of protruded disc and shortly afterwards, in 1858, Luschka described it more fully. At autopsy Luschka found a soft greyish knob of tissue on the surface of the posterior longitudinal ligament between L2 and L3; on sectioning the disc horizontally he found that this tissue had arisen from the nucleus pulposus that had burst through the annulus. He postulated that if this mass continued to expand it could burst through the ligament and cause cord compression. In 1896 Kocher found a high disc protusion in the course of an autopsy on a man who had fallen 100 feet.

In 1911 two classic papers appeared, one from Glasgow and the other from Boston. The Glasgow paper describes a man who died from a traumatic paraplegia and was found to have a massive disc prolapse. Goldthwait's paper from Boston discusses a man who developed a paraplegia after a spinal manipulation for back pain (a warning to all). He theorises on the basis of this and produces a speculative description of lumbo-sacral instability as a cause of lumbago and sciatica. Amongst other ideas, he thought that a disc prolapse could cause cord and root pressure. He includes a drawing of this notion, which is so accurate that it could be used in a textbook today.

These papers did not attract much attention. Surgeons had by this time started to operate on the spinal cord with increasing frequency, but regarded disc protrusions as sessile chondromata or fibromata.

In the twenties Schmorl and his school were studying the spinal column as a routine during autopsies and found disc protrusions in about 15 per cent. of autopsies. In the later twenties "chondromata" were a fairly commonplace finding for the neurosurgeon. However it was not until 1934 that Mixter and Barr established firstly the fact that these chondromata were in fact disc prolapses and secondly the connection between sciatica and disc protusion. These two surgeons from Massachusetts General Hospital described 19 cases which they had operated on: 4 cervical discs, 4 thoracic, 10 lumbar and 1 sacral. They ended their paper with these words, "I think fusion should be combined with operation where there is any question of an unstable spine, and I believe that a ruptured disc may be unstable".

At first the prolapse was removed by full transdural laminectomy but within a few years, in 1939, Love had evolved the interlaminar approach which did not require the removal of any bone. After the Second World War disc surgery was very popular but did not prove to be a panacea for sciatica and today a more conservative mood prevails.

Domenico Cotugno (or Cotunnius), 1736-1822

Cotugno was born in Ruvo, Italy; his father, not rich, spared nothing to give his son a good education. This appears to have been a wise decision. At the age of 9 years Domenico could speak the Latin tongue with fluency; at the age of 18 he was elected to the position of Physician at the Hospital for Incurables at Naples—perhaps it was considered a safe appointment for a teenager. By the age of 20 he became Professor of Surgery at the Hospital and occupied the chair for sixty-six years until his death aged 86.

He is remembered for his discovery of the cerebrospinal fluid in normal animals, his discovery of the aqueducts of the inner ear, his descriptions of sciatica, typhoid ulcers, and the presence of material that coagulated on heating the urine of patients with acute nephritis.

On his deathbed he left 100,000 ducats to the hospital he had served so long.

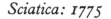

Sciatica: 1775

A Treatise on the Nervous Sciatica or Nervous Hip Gout

by Dominicus Cotunnius, PHIL. & MED.D.

1. It is a thing very well known amongst physicians, that the name *Sciatica* is given to that species of pain which seizes the hips about those parts where the thigh-bones form the joints; a pain seldom felt in both, but often in one, so as to render the patient lame on that side which it invests. This name is of Greek origin, and is derived from the seat of the disorder; for the hip in Greek is called ἰσχίον but I much doubt whether it was adopted by the Latins before the time of *Pliny* the elder. For altho' *Cato* has the word *Ischiacos*, yet *Celsus*, who was very accurate in his knowledge of the Latin names, which were affixed in his time to diseases, when he has occasion to mention this pain, chuses to call it *Dolor Coxae*.

2. The species of the Sciatica are various, according to the various parts in which the pain is felt; and altho', as hitherto, physicians have not discriminated between them so accurately as they ought; yet every one is separately to be distinguished and marked out by its characteristic symptoms, as each demands its proper treatment in the cure. The principal species of Sciatica that deserve our attention are two; one, where the pain is fixed in the hip, and extends no further; the other, where it runs along, as it were, in a track, and is propagated even down the foot, on the same side. Although, in the *former*, it is not only one part of the hip that is always affected, nor the pain produced always by the same cause; yet because it is generally felt about the joint, I think it would be properly termed the *arthritic Sciatica*. The *latter*, because it has its situation in the nerves which run along the hip (notwithstanding it is by some called the *true*, as by *Prosperus Martianus* and by others the *bastard Sciatica*, as by *Riolanus*) I am of opinion ought to be called the *Nervous Sciatica*.

3. At present, I shall leave the *Arthritic Sciatica* out of the question. For I know very well that many very eminent men who have gone before me, have left nothing for me to say, either on its various causes, or various situations; to witness, those very excellent physicians *Morgagni*, and *Antony de Haen*. I shall take upon me to speak only of the *Nervous Sciatica*, the principal causes of which lie as yet buried in obscurity. But I shall divide this Sciatica into two species. The one is a fixed pain in the hip, situated chiefly behind the great trochanter of the thigh, and extends itself upwards to the Os sacrum, and downwards by the exterior side of the thigh even to the knee; this pain seldom stops at the knee, but often runs on the exterior part of the head of the *Fibula*, and descends to the fore part of the leg, where it pursues its course along the outside of the anterior spine of the Tibia, before the exterior ancle, and so ends on the Dorsum Pedis. The other is fixed pain in the groin, which runs along inside of the thigh and leg. The *former*, as it is situated in the posterior part of the hip, and arises from an affection of the *Ischiadic Nerve*, I shall call the *Posterior Nervous Sciatica*: the latter, which invests the fore part of the hip, and is propagated along the *Crural Nerve*, I shall term the *Anterior Nervous Sciatica*. I shall now, as briefly as I can, relate what discoveries and observations I have made, and what judgment I have formed on these two species of the disease.

4. To begin with the *Posterior Sciatica Nervosa*. I have observed that it is either *continual* or *intermitting*: sometimes it tortures the patient day and night, without any intermission; but more commonly remits now and then, and returns again at stated intervals. But it is common to both, to have the pains exacerbated in the evening; and the *intermitting Sciatica* generally begins its attacks at that time. In the attacks, the convulsion of the part is so great, that the patient is tortured with a sensation like the cramp, leaps out of bed, as the warmth there increases it, and flies to the open air for relief. In the beginning, this Sciatica is almost always continual, and intermits by degrees, as if it was tired. This intermitting, however, is oftentimes by far the most excruciating torture, and seems to pause from one attack, to collect and increase all its strength for the next. But, as I have known many persons, who, from suffering a continual, have been attacked by an intermitting, I never once saw the reverse, or observed the continual preceded by the intermitting Sciatica; for, then the disease would abate instead of increasing, and the first attack be the most violent. However this may be; if the disorder remains a long time uncured, a *Semiparalysis* of the affected part will be the consequence, which is always accompanied with a great emaciation; and an insuperable lameness. From all the examples I can collect, I never saw a perfect palsy produced by this Sciatica.

5. As I observed all the symptoms accurately, I concluded the judgment I had formed was right; and that it consisted in an affection of the *Ischiadic Nerve*. Though chance has never thrown an opportunity in my way to prove this by the dissection of any

person who died in this disorder, I do not in the least imagine that I am assuming a dubious state of the case, in pointing out its seat. For in this particular I am very well satisfied both by my own diligent observations of the symptoms, as well as by the happy and absolute cures I have performed in consequence of them. If I am here deceived, I am happily deceived, and I am not very solicitous to be delivered from the infatuation, since in it I have such success with my patients. By the way, I think the physician, who after having diligently examined into the situation, and effects of the disorder, should deny that affection of the Ischiadic Nerves, could understand but little of the fabric of the human body. For as to what relates to the seat of the disorder, this is so clear, that if the patient will but point out with his finger the track of the pain from the *Os sacrum* to the foot, we shall find him, like a skilful anatomist, tracing out the exact progress of the Ischiadic Nerve. That Hippocrates, from the track of the pain, calls it an affection of the crural vein, is excusable, by reason of the ignorance of those times respecting the nerves: and that *Martianus*, after those learned men, *Joannes Riolanus* and *Fernelius*, had professed the truth, followed this opinion of Hippocrates, must be attributed to his ignorance of the circulation of the blood. For as he observed, in a certain mason who was his patient in this disorder, that in the exacerbation of the pain, which happened in the paroxysms, all the veins that branched along the outside of the affected hip and leg swelled and puffed up wonderfully, and immediately upon the pain subsiding, totally disappeared, he concluded, that this manifestly proved the descent of the morbific matter by the veins of the leg. If he had known that it was impossible for the veins to be the conductors of the matter, and that the muscles of the affected part were so convulsed as to puff out the external lax veins by the constrained opposite course of the blood, he might have indeed been taught that this phenomenon could not in any shape prove this opinion of Hippocrates.

6. Not only the situation and track of the pain demonstrate that the seat of the disorder is in the Ischiadic Nerve, but likewise the various affections which follow prove it clearly. For the insuperable lameness that is sometimes the consequence of it, shews, that the powers of the muscles in moving the thigh and leg are weakened: but the power of those muscles that maintain the free motion of the nerves, are not commonly weakened for a long time. For a Semi-palsy coming on, gives us a striking proof that the nerves are affected. It is usually accompanied with an emaciation, which distinguishes the torpor of the limbs arising from long inactivity, from that impotence which is brought on by wounding the nerves. Therefore, if the nerves of the hip in this Sciatica are affected, I do not see how it can be doubted that the Ischiadic, of all the nerves traversing the hips, as the pain is fixed there, is not the cause and seat of the disorder. In this nerve the pain is felt, in this nerve we are to search for the cause of lameness, and from its affection the origin of the *Semiparalysis* and *Tabes*.

The cause of sciatica

He drew attention to the cerebrospinal fluid circulating in the dural sacs. He thought this could be present in excessive amounts diffusing into the peripheral nerves.

32. Since, therefore, an abundant, or acrid fluid, abiding in the outer Vaginae of the Ischiadic Nerve, may cause the Posterior Nervous Sciatica, let us now see how it generates all the symptoms and effects of it. In the first place, if it arises from too great an abundance of fluid, the Vaginae of the nerves will consequently be strained, and the enclosed nervous filaments compressed, so that the leg will be rather benumbed than painful. On the other hand, if the fluid be acrid, then the pain will be sharp and permanent. But from whichsoever of these causes it arises, the pains will be exacerbated towards the evening; for at that time a man's body grows warm, and the pain is increased, either by the more rapid circulation of the blood's causing a greater quantity of fluid to be thrown into the Vaginae; or by the increased heat's exciting or adding a greater stimulus to the acrid matter. The pain that the patient suffers in this exacerbation, can hardly be expressed.

Cotunnius goes on to compare sciatica with brachial neuralgia.

31. I now flatter myself that I have produced some probable reasons, and causes, of the generation of pain in the Ischiadic Nerve; and why its trunk and branch, which descends to the leg, feel the track of the pain and are more adapted to receive the causes, than the other nerves of the body, except the Cubital. Nor is there here any room to cavil at me, because the Cubital Nerve has almost the same disposition, and yet is seldomer affected with pain. For, although this may be owing to the Cubital Nerve's having but a small track uncovered with muscles, the pain is not so rare to be met with as is imagined. Indeed, I have often known the Cubital affected at the same time with the Ischiadic Nerve; and especially when the cause of the pain was internal, and might be communicated to both nerves. This consent, and agreement of pain in the elbow and hip, have been observed by me more than once, in curing those who were harrassed with a rheumatic or venereal Virus; and I do not doubt, but that, if anyone would attend to it, we should frequently observe an alliance between these two pains. Nay, as I have often observed, the pain of the hips descend by degrees to the foot, or rise from the foot to the hip, I have in like manner found the pain of the elbow ascend to the shoulder, and reach to the extremities of the fingers. There is so great a similarity and consent between these pains, whether we regard the disposition of the affected parts, or the nature of the pain, that I think Celsus, in judging these two pains, has done right to couple them together, and even put them upon a par. Indeed, if the name of the Sciatica had not taken its origin from the seat of the pain, but from its appearance, I myself

should not hesitate to call that pain of the arm, the *Nervous Cubital Sciatica*; for it agrees with the Posterior Nervous Sciatica, in appearance, situation, symptoms, and cure.

George Stevenson Middleton, 1853-1928

George Middleton was born in Aberdeen and graduated from Glasgow. Later as a physician he joined the teaching staff and instituted a post-graduate class on Sundays, probably initiating post-graduate education in Glasgow. His writings were mainly descriptions of unusual and interesting cases.

John Hammond Teacher, 1869-1930

Teacher was a graduate of Glasgow University who became Professor of Pathology. His main interest was in gynaecological pathology, and he achieved fame for describing a very early foetus.

Injury of the Spinal Cord due to Rupture of an Intervertebral Disc during Muscular Effort

by George S. Middleton, M.D., and John H. Teacher, M.D., 1911

The following case is of interest, because it seems to throw light upon certain cases of spinal myelitis and haemorrhage into the spinal cord arising out of strains and racks of the back in men engaged upon heavy work. So far as we are aware, the lesion is one which has not hitherto been observed, as we have been unable, after considerable search in literature and enquiry among pathologists and surgeons, to find any record of an exactly similar case.

Summary—A man was lifting a heavy plate from the floor to a bench, when he felt a "crack" in the small of his back. He suffered intense pain, and was unable to straighten himself. Paraplegia soon developed, and patient died sixteen days later, principally from the effects of bedsores and septic cystitis. The cause of the paraplegia was haemorrhage and softening in the lumbar enlargement of the spinal cord, and the cause of this was found in a mass of the pulp of an intervertebral disc which had been displaced into the vertebral canal.

With regard to the mechanism of the injury, it can be inferred from the history of the case that the man, at the moment at which he felt the "crack" in his back must have had his back more or less bent forward, with the lumbar and abdominal muscles in full action.

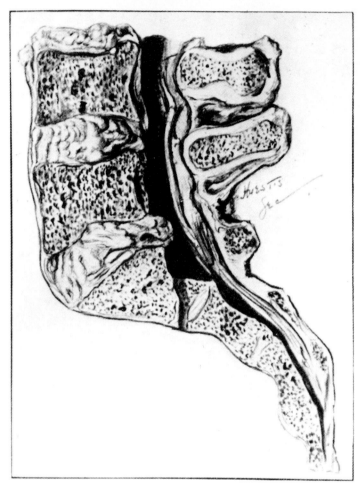

Goldthwait: Prolapsed Intervertebral Disc

This would cause powerful compression of the intervertebral discs, with the anterior margins of the vertebrae approximated to one another, and, therefore, in a favourable position for displacement of the pulp of the intervertebral disc backwards, if that were possible.

To test this theory of the injury experiments were made to see whether the pulp of the intervertebral disc could be squeezed out through the strong surrounding ligaments, and the direction which it would take.

In one a successful result was obtained. The first three lumbar vertebrae from the body of a well-developed man with no disease of the column were placed in a carpenter's wooden vice, and pressure made rather more to the front than to the back. The cord and the nerves had been cut out, leaving the dura *in situ*. It was noted before pressure that the position of the intervertebral discs was shown by a slight bulging inwards. After pressure had been applied a definite rounded prominence could be seen opposite the disc between the first and second lumbar vertebrae, close to the side of the posterior longitudinal ligament.

The pressure had not been very powerful—certainly not enough to crush the bones at all. Repeating the experiment with more powerful pressure the swelling was seen to increase slightly.

The arches were then cut out and the dura mater raised. The rounded swelling was found with the fibrous outer layer of the disc intact. Pressure with an iron vice to crushing of the bone failed to produce any further swelling.

On cutting through the disc with a sharp knife it was found that the swelling actually was due to displacement of the soft pulp, which had forced its way through the inner fibrous layers of the disc as far as the outer sheath. The corresponding area on the other side was unchanged. The pulp of the disc had, therefore, been displaced, and it had travelled in the direction which it must have followed in the victim of the accident.

Joel Goldthwait, 1866-1961

Goldthwait was born in Marblehead, Massachusetts. He planned to work in scientific agriculture and graduated, but after one unhappy day in business, he decided to try something else. He graduated again in medicine from Harvard in 1890. He worked for an orthopaedic surgeon and made this his speciality. At the turn of the century there were no hospital facilities in Boston for the crippled and disabled over the age of 12. As a result of agitation he acquired a third floor room to work from, and the success of this led to an orthopaedic out-patient clinic being formed at Massachusetts General Hospital. He raised funds to build a ward which was opened in

1909 and he became its first head. A little later he published his article on the importance of the lumbo-sacral joint. Later he organised a school of physical education and another for occupational therapy students, in addition to his great activity writing and teaching. During his life he was at the forefront of the American orthopaedic scene and played a major rôle in the development of the Boston school of orthopaedics.

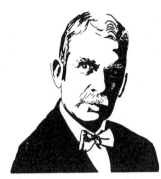

The Lumbo-Sacral Articulation. An Explanation of Many Cases of "Lumbago", "Sciatica" and Paraplegia

by Joel E. Goldthwait, M.D., Boston, 1911

An experience of the writer within the past year in connection with the treatment of a patient with a spinal lesion was so disastrous to the patient and so distressing to the writer that a series of investigations were started in the hope of bringing some relief to the patient and at the same time of preventing such happenings in the future. It is this study which represents the basis of this communication, and in order that it may be fully understood the case that led to it is first reported.

Goldthwait described a 39-year-old man who strained his back. A displacement of the right sacro-iliac joint was diagnosed and replaced under anaesthesia. He made a normal recovery but three months later his pain recurred and a strain of both sacro-iliacs was diagnosed. The following day he felt something 'slip' in his back as he leaned forward to get out of a bath. It produced sudden severe pain; his body was drawn forwards and to one side and the pain radiated into the legs. Goldthwait manipulated his sacro-iliac joint under anaesthesia but without relief so later in the day he started to put on a plaster jacket in hypertension. While he was doing so the patient had another severe pain and within a few minutes developed a motor and sensory paraplegia with paralysis of the sphincters. When he was put on his side this disappeared but returned when he turned over in bed. By the following morning the paraplegia was complete and remained so.

After six weeks Harvey Cushing explored the spinal canal from L1 to S3 but found no abnormality. The patient improved somewhat and eight months later was able to move with sticks.

Goldthwait's powers of reasoning were stimulated. He thought that this cauda equina lesion had occurred at the lumbosacral level because of clicks from this region, tenderness and the pattern of paralysis. He studied the anatomy and abnormalities of the region, and suggested that the lumbosacral joint could become subluxated by the transverse process of L5 striking the sacral ala and prising the joint open. He mentions that Dr. A. H. Crosbie had seen, but not published, a case of paraplegia due to proven disc prolapse. The illustration gives his impression of what it would look like.

It is a paper that covers possibilities; because in view of the negative laminectomy, he had no evidence to incriminate a massive disc prolapse which would today seem the most likely cause of his patient's troubles.

Here are his final conclusions.

> The lumbo-sacral articulation varies very greatly in its stability, depending upon peculiarities in the formation of the articular processes and of the transverse processes; that these peculiarities not only result in less than the normal strength of the joint, but may represent mechanical elements which not only produce strain and cause pain but may lead to such great instability that actual displacement of the bones may result, with at the same time the separation of the posterior portion of the intervertebral disk.
>
> In such displacement, if the fifth lumbar slides forward upon the sacrum, spondylolisthesis, the condition is usually compensated for, and pressure upon the cauda equina or the nerve roots does not occur.
>
> If the displacement be upon one side, the spine must be rotated and the articular process of the fifth is drawn into the spinal canal with such narrowing that paraplegia may result, or the crowding backward of the intervertebral disk alone may be so great as to cause paraplegia, but of more gradual development.
>
> Weakness of the joints or the partial displacements may cause irritation of the nerves inside or outside of the canal and produce the bilateral leg pains often called sciatica.

Morton's Metatarsalgia: Thomas G. Morton, 1835-1903

Morton was born in Philadelphia in 1835, the son of a physician, and graduated from the University of Pennsylvania in 1856 with a thesis on Cataract. He stayed on at the Hospital for three years and was elected to the staff in 1864. He made his name as a teacher and as a daring and original operator. In April 1887 he performed perhaps the first successful laparotomy for acute appendicitis; he did this after losing a son and a brother from this condition having vainly tried to persuade a surgeon to operate. He also worked at an eye hospital and collaborated with Weir Mitchell.

During the Civil War he worked as surgeon at Chestnut Hill, and showed great energy establishing military hospitals. After the war he founded the Philadelphia Orthopaedic Hospital.

He died of cholera in Philadelphia.

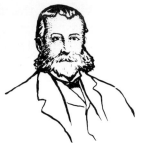

A Peculiar and Painful Affection of the Fourth Metatarso-Phalangeal Articulation

by Thomas G. Morton, M.D., 1876

one of the Surgeons to the Pennsylvania Hospital, Surgeon to the Philadelphia Orthopaedic Hospital, etc.

During the past few years, I have had under my care a number of cases of a peculiar and painful affection of the foot, which, so far as I am aware, has not been described.

In these cases the pain has been localized in the fourth metatarsophalangeal articulation; in several instances it followed at once after an injury of the foot, in others it was gradually developed from pressure, while in others there was no recognized cause.

Case 1: Mrs. J., the mother of three children, consulted me in July, 1870, and gave the following history of her case:-

"During the summer of 1868, while travelling in Switzerland, I made a pedestrian tour to the Valley of the Faulhorn Mountain, and when descending a steep ravine, I trod upon quite a large stone which rolled from under my foot, causing me to slip, throwing my entire weight upon the forward foot; though not falling, I found my right foot injured; the pain was intense and accompanied by fainting sensations. With considerable difficulty I reached the valley of the Grindenwald, where for hours I endured great suffering. After this I found it impossible to wear a shoe even for a few moments, the least pressure inducing an attack of severe pain. At no time did the foot or toe swell or present any evidence of having been injured. During the succeeding five years the foot was never entirely free from pain, often my suffering has been very severe, and coming on in paroxysms. I have been able only to wear a very large shoe, and only for a limited space of time, invariably being obliged to remove it every half hour or so, to relieve the foot. Much of the time I have gone without any covering except a stocking, and even at nights have suffered intensely; slight pressure of the finger on the tender spot causes the same sensation as wearing a shoe. During the past year or so I have walked but little, and have consequently suffered much less."

In this case, succeeding a contusion of the foot, acute pain came on, which continued for several hours. This was followed by permanent local sensitiveness, increased to absolute pain with the slightest pressure of a shoe, or even sock; and at times, without any pressure or known cause, there would come on paroxysms of excessive pain. The neuralgia was always referred to the metatarsophalangeal joint of the fourth toe; during the severe paroxysms it extended, occasionally, to the knee. There was neither redness nor swelling anywhere about the foot. The head of the fourth metatarsal, with the phalangeal base, and the soft parts about the joint, were exceedingly sensitive. From the entire absence of all inflammatory symptoms, it seemed as if there might be, to account for the severity of the paroxysms, either a neuroma or some nerve hypertrophy. This sensitive condition was constantly aggravated by the almost unavoidable pressure of the very movable fifth metatarsal and little toe upon the fourth metatarso-phalangeal joint. A deep excavation in the sole of a broad shoe, corresponding to the joint of the fourth toe, was recommended; this with varied anodyne applications to the part gave no marked relief. The least pressure of a shoe, and sometimes even that of a stocking, produced a recurrence of intense pain. The patient was of a nervous temperament, with a predisposition to pulmonary disease, and was not in a condition to undergo any treatment which would confine her to the house. In June, 1873, I saw Mrs. J., again; then in consultation; there had been during this interval no improvement. A short time before seeing this patient the second time, I had under my care another case which presented the same form of neuralgia, which followed an injury, and was successfully treated by an excision of the fourth metatarso-phalangeal joint.

The joint of the fifth metatarsal being so much posterior to that of the fourth, the base of the first phalanx of the little toe is brought on a line with the head and neck of the fourth metatarsal, and the head of the fifth opposite the neck of the fourth.

There is very slight lateral motion in the first three metatarsal bones, on account of their peculiar tarsal articulations; this is not so with the fourth and the fifth, which have much greater mobility, the fifth considerably much more than the fourth, and in this respect it resembles the fifth metacarpal. It will be found that lateral pressure brings the head of the fifth metatarsal and the little toe into direct contact with the base of the first phalanx, and head and neck of the fourth, and to some extent the extremity of the fifth metatarsal rolls above and under this bone.

The external plantar nerve gives off superficial and deep muscular branches, the superficial branch separates into two digital nerves, which supply the outer and inner side of the fifth toe, and the outer side of the fourth; small branches are distributed freely between the fourth and fifth toes, about the metatarso-phalangeal joints.

To the peculiar position which the fourth metatarso-phalangeal articulation bears to that of the fifth, the great mobility of the fifth metatarsal, which by lateral pressure is brought into contact with the fourth, and lastly, the proximity of the digital branches of the external plantar nerve, which are, under certain circumstances, liable to be bruised by, or pinched between the fourth and fifth metatarsals, may be ascribed the neuralgia in this region.

In chronic cases, such as have been described, no other treatment except complete excision of the irritable metatarso-phalangeal joint with the surrounding soft parts will be likely to prove permanently successful.

Although Morton was unaware of a description of plantar neuralgia, the condition had in fact been observed by the royal chiropodist. Lewis

Durlacher, Surgeon Chiropodist to the Queen, wrote a Treatise on Corns, Bunions, the Diseases of nails, and the General Management of the Feet, in 1845. In addition to describing George IV's ingrowing toenail which he cared for, he described plantar neuralgia.

> It is a kind of neuralgia seated between the toes, but which fortunately is not very common. It constitutes a most troublesome and severe complaint, and one very difficult of removal.
>
> The patient complains of a severe pain between two of the toes, along the inside of one or the other, generally the second and third, he can seldom tell which; it extends up the leg, and is increased when the toes are pressed together, more particularly after walking. Notwithstanding the most careful examination of the part, no obvious cause can be discovered for the pain, and like all similar affections of the nerves, there is not any remedy to be depended upon, as it appears to defy all normal medical treatment.
>
> Another form of neuralgic affection occasionally attacks the plantar nerve on the sole of the foot, between the third and fourth metetarsal bones, but nearest to the third, and close to the articulation with the phalanx. The spot where the pain is experienced can at all times be exactly covered by the finger. The pain which cannot be produced by the mere pressure of the finger, becomes very severe while walking, or whenever the foot is put to the ground.
>
> The complaint appears to me to be very similar to that which I have just described, and I cannot assign any cause for its occurrence. Relief can only be afforded by the application of lateral compression, a strip of plaster about an inch wide being drawn tightly over the foot and round the sole. I believe this application acts by drawing the metatarsal bones closer, and thus affording protection to the affected nerve, which, when the parts are capable of expansion, is more exposed to pressure.

Carpal Tunnel Syndrome

Paget was apparently the first in 1853 to realise that the median nerve could be compressed at the wrist. Later, in 1883, Ormerod described the typical, clinical picture of the condition but had no idea of its aetiology.

Reports similar to his appeared sporadically. In 1913 Pierre Marie and Foix demonstrated at autopsy in a case with bilateral thenar atrophy that the median nerve was compressed as it passed through the carpal tunnel.

Woltman in 1941 reported perhaps the first case treated surgically and Seddon operated on two cases in 1945. Russell Brain in 1947 wrote in the *Lancet* about 14 cases, of which six were treated surgically, and it was soon after this that a patient with carpal tunnel syndrome stood a chance of having it recognised and treated. Now it is one of the most commonly performed operations on the hand.

Median Nerve Compression: Paget, 1853

Mr. Hilton has told me this case:

> A man was at Guy's Hospital, who, in consequence of a fracture at the lower end of the radius, repaired by an excessive quantity of new bone, suffered compression of the median nerve. He had ulceration of the thumb and fore and middle fingers, which resisted various treatment, and was only cured by so binding the wrist that, the parts on the palmar aspect being relaxed, the pressure on the nerve was removed. So long as this was done, the ulcers became and remained well; but as soon as the man was allowed to use his hand, the pressure on the nerves was renewed, and the ulceration of the parts supplied by them returned.

Joseph Arderne Ormerod, 1848-1925

The son of an Archdeacon of Suffolk, Joseph Ormerod was born at Starston, Norfolk and came from a distinguished medical family. He trained at St. Bartholomew's Hospital, graduating in 1875. He was a neurologist by inclination, and was unlucky enough to strike a bad patch at Bart's—everyone wanted to get on the medical staff. He became an early version of a time-expired Registrar: at the age of 45, he became Assistant Physician, and was only a full physician for nine years before he had to retire under the age limit.

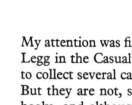

On a Peculiar Numbness and Paresis of the Hands

by J. A. Ormerod, 1883

My attention was first called to this set of symptoms by Dr. Wickham Legg in the Casualty Department. Since that time I have been able to collect several cases, and they are, I am sure, sufficiently common. But they are not, so far as I know, described in most medical text-books, and although in no sense grave, yet they may be sufficiently troublesome to cause the patient to relinquish her employment. I hope, therefore, that the following examples may not be thought altogether uninteresting.

The symptoms are remarkably definite in character. They occur in women, usually about the climacteric age, and begin in the night. On waking, the patient has a feeling in the hands, or hands and arms (commonly of both sides), of numbness, deadness, pins and needles; sometimes there is actual pain, severe enough to wake her. There is also loss of power; the hands and arms become useless, and she cannot hold things. This may so far predominate that the patient comes to be treated for a supposed paralysis. Sometimes also the patients say that the hands swell, the veins swell, &c., at the time.

The symptoms pass off in a little time, and rubbing suggests itself as a natural remedy. But occasionally they manifest themselves in the daytime also, and then principally when the patient sets about her ordinary work—washing, scrubbing, needlework, &c.

I.—February 1882.—Mrs. S., age between 50 and 60, an active and healthy woman, has had for the past eighteen months the following symptoms:-

She is woke up nightly by pains in the fingers, hands and up the fore-arms. The hands seem to become stiff and useless, and when she gets up look, she says, as if they were dead. The pain is severe and prevents sleep.

She is (just now) rather pale and puffy looking.

Pulse a little hard, and second sound over aorta rather accentuated. No albuminuria. On the articular ends of some of the phalanges (right hand) are small hard nodules. She says that the fingers are rather stiff through rheumatism.

She took iodide of potassium for a fortnight with no benefit; colchicum tried for a few nights did not suit her at all; quassia and iron taken for over a fortnight gave only slight and temporary relief. A fresh nodule appeared on the distal end of the middle phalanx of the left hand; it was (at least while forming) larger and less hard than the others, though firm.

She connected her complaint with the use of water for scrubbing floors; gave up her place as servant on this account, and her hands improved afterwards.

This patient (whom I have had ample opportunities of seeing) was not at all hysterical, and there was no neurosis in her family.

Myositis Ossificans Progressiva: John Freke, 1688-1756

John Freke was born in London and was apprenticed to Mr. Richard Blundell, marrying his daughter. In 1729 he joined the staff of St. Bartholomew's Hospital, and in the same year became F.R.S. He suffered from gout, which forced him to retire from the hospital in 1755. He was a man of wide culture, well known in literary circles: he was a friend of Fielding who mentioned him in *Tom Jones*.

Myositis Ossificans Progressiva: Freke, 1740

(*Extract from a letter to the Royal Society*)

Yesterday there came a boy of healthy look, and about fourteen years old, to ask of us at the Hospital, what should be done to cure him of many large Swellings on the Back, which began about Three Years since, and have continued to grow as large on many Parts as a

Penny-loaf, particularly on the Left Side: they arise from all the *vertebrae* of the Neck, and reach down to the *os sacrum*; they likewise arise from every Rib of his body, and joining together in all Parts of his Back, as the Ramifications of Coral do, they made, as it were, a fixed Bony Pair of Bodices.

If this be found worthy your Thoughts it will afford a Pleasure to Gentlemen,

Yours Most Humble Servant,

John Freke.

It is to be observed that he had no other symptoms of rickets in any joint of his limbs.

5 OSTEOCHONDRITIS JUVENALIS

Osteochondritis Juvenalis

This disorder, which includes a great variety of different lesions, probably of different aetiology, was not clearly distinguished until the coming of X-rays. Osgood seems to have described the first lesion in 1903. In the next 25 years a rush of articles appeared from different countries; some of them were synchronous so that double- and triple-barrelled eponyms are common —for example osteochondritis of the femoral head was described in 1910 in three different languages by Legg, Calvé, and Perthes.

For those attracted to osteochondritismanship here are some names attached to its rarer forms:

Sternal end of clavicle	—	Friedrich
Internal epicondyle of humerus	—	Legg
Capitulum of humerus	—	Panner
Olecranon	—	Mouchet
Heads of metacarpal bones	—	Mauclaire
Iliac crests	—	Buchman
Ischial tuberosity	—	Voltancoli
Upper end of tibia	—	Ritter
Sesamoids of big toe	—	Trèves

Scheuermann's Disease: Holger Werfel Scheuermann, 1877-1960

The son of a Danish doctor, Scheuermann trained in orthopaedics and radiology. In 1935 he became chief radiologist at the Cripple's Hospital and was the best known radiologist in Denmark.

He described juvenile kyphosis in 1921, and presented a thesis on this subject to the university for his doctorate. They would not accept it. Finally at the age of 80 he was granted an honorary doctorate in recognition of his work.

Clearly Scheuerman was not the first to recognise this condition as a description written in 1826 shows. He did however, recognise the cause of the deformity.

74

The Stoop or Semi-circular Curve Forwards: R. A. Stafford, 1832

Nothing is more common than to see a weakly, over-grown boy, about fourteen or fifteen years of age, stooping forwards, as if he would fall at every step he takes. The poor lad is blamed, both by his parents and school master, and is laughed at by his companions, for so careless a habit. The fact, however, is, that the muscles of his back are so weak that they have not sufficient strength to support him. In spite, therefore, of all remonstrances, he still stoops, and, vexed at constant reproofs, he seeks, by lolling in all directions, to relieve himself, till at length he falls into bad habits, and the deformity becomes confirmed.

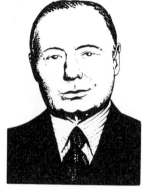

Kyphosis Dorsalis Juvenalis: H. Scheuermann, 1921

It is possible to distinguish a group of cases amongst the curvatures of the spine which begin during puberty that are morphologically different from the rest and have other features in common which command interest.

The type to be discussed below is the dorsal kyphosis—a genuine sagittal curve due to a fixed curvature of the vertebral column and distinct from a round back, an error of posture, which can be actively corrected in whole or in part.

He describes a series of 105 such patients in whom the curvature was purely sagittal in 60 and accompanied by slight lateral deviation in 45. The peak incidence was at the age of 16, and 88 per cent. of the cases were males.

> At first sight it seems that puberty, a period of rapid growth culminating at about the age of 16, must be an important factor. The case histories of most of these patients reveal that the deformity of the back followed manual work of some kind. The agricultural workers are in the absolute majority and most of them state that the curvature of the spine developed slowly over the course of six months or a year, often accompanied by pain in the back which radiated to the sides, and all the patients stated that the pain definitely disappeared on lying down.

Scheuermann notes that the patients were generally quite well built and muscular, and that they themselves do not notice any deformity; it is usually their friends who tell them that their backs are curved. There were no neurological signs. He has never seen this curvature develop in the neck or in the lumbar area.

Scheuermann's view was that though age and occupation must be regarded as important, heavy loads are not always the cause because it was found in people who had not carried out heavy work. It was not due to paralysis of muscle, and the deformity was in the vertebral column. Radiographs showed nothing abnormal with a patient lying recumbent, because of the superimposition of the vertebrae. Only lateral pictures, though technically difficult at that time, gave some information.

An X-ray picture in a recent case (i.e. during the first six months) of a typical dorsal kyphosis shows that the vertebrae which lie at the most concave portion of the curvature are considerably narrower anteriorly than posteriorly. The vertebrae become wedge-shaped. The epiphysis is no longer triangular but becomes broad and irregular; the vertebrae are also irregular, which points to abnormal conditions in the line of growth. The further away from the curvature, the more normal the vertebrae become. In Scheuermann's X-rays there are only three vertebrae affected.

He wondered whether the kyphosis caused the wedging or whether the wedging caused the kyphosis, but he came to the conclusion that the primary cause must lie in the growing area between the epiphysis and the body of the vertebrae.

> Everyone looking at these X-rays has to admit that there is some abnormality. There is such a big difference between the profile of the growth line of the body of a normal dorsal vertebrae and one of these affected vertebrae. The wedge shape has arisen because the vertebra has become smaller in these areas while the intervertebral discs remain unchanged.

He points out that radiographs taken at a later stage do not show this broad epiphyseal plate any more. He compares the epiphyseal changes with the clinical course of osteochondritis at various sites and concludes that this is a related condition, and should be called osteochondritis deformans juvenilis dorsi. He noted that it occurred in horses and that effective therapy is unknown. If the pain is severe, he suggested one to two weeks in bed; plaster of Paris dressing or suspensions in lordosis were tried as well as physiotherapy and massage, but were ineffective.

"The deformity will remain despite any treatment known."

Coxa Plana

For many years this condition was confused with tuberculosis and yielded outstanding results with treatment. Today it is one of the few orthopaedic conditions for which prolonged bed rest, reminiscent of the treatment of tuberculosis during the last century, is still advocated.

It was recognised independently by three surgeons who published their papers in the same year—Legg in February 1910, Calvé in July, and Perthes in October. They were very magnanimous and in subsequent articles gave the credit to each other. Georg Perthes pointed out that Legg had lectured on the topic a year before (Perthes, 1920) and Legg wrote that it was largely due to the work of Perthes that the condition was being recognised (Legg, 1916).

Arthur T. Legg, 1874-1939

Born at Chelsea, Massachusetts, Arthur Legg graduated from Harvard in 1900. Receiving his orthopaedic training at Boston, he slowly moved up in the hierarchy. He pioneered with Goldthwait the first adult orthopaedic clinic at Boston. After many years as a self sufficient bachelor, he married the nursing sister of the private ward in 1936.

He is best known for his descriptions of coxa plana, on which he wrote eight papers, but had other wide interests.

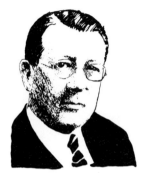

An Obscure Affection of the Hip-Joint: 1910

by Arthur T. Legg, M.D., Boston, Mass.
Junior Assistant Surgeon, Children's Hospital

We are at times painfully aware of the fact that there are many symptoms which we readily recognise in our clinical observations to which we can assign no cause, and it is also an undoubted fact that there are many conditions even which exist today of which we are ignorant, simply from our neglect to observe, or from faulty observation, or, again, from faulty deduction even from good observation.

The cases which I bring to your attention today seem to me illustrative of the fact that we, in the past, have not observed certain conditions which truly exist, and that now, having observed, we naturally must ask ourselves, are our observations faulty or are they correct? and, assuming them to be correct, what is the cause of the condition?

The first case, a well-developed girl of eight, was brought to the Children's Hospital in October, 1907, with a history of a fall nine months before, immediately followed by a limp on the right which had persisted. There had been no pain or constitutional symptoms.

Examination showed normal flexion of the right hip with all other motions much limited. There was very slight spasm, slight atrophy of the thigh and calf, but no shortening. There was a slight amount of thickening anterior to the neck. The motions of the left hip were normal.

A traction hip splint was applied, which she has worn since. She has had no acute symptoms, nor pain, and has remained in excellent general condition. The very slight spasm present at the first examination disappeared in about a month.

Examination of the right hip at the present time shows motion in flexion to 100°, abduction to 50°, adduction normal. Internal and external rotation is possible to about 45°. The thickening about the joint has remained the same, and the right leg now measures one quarter of an inch longer than the left.

There has been no pain or limp on the left, and the motions of this hip are normal. A slight amount of thickening, however, is felt about this hip.

The Von Pirquet test was negative. Roentgenological examination shows the head of the right femur to be flattened and apparently spread out. The neck appears thickened and shorter than normal. An area of increased radiability appears in the upper part of the head and neck. The left or apparently normal side shows the same condition with the exception of the area of increased radiability.

He describes four further cases.

In reviewing the cases, the following facts in a general way are observed:

(1) Age, five to eight years.

(2) History of injury.

(3) Limp.

(4) Thickening about the neck of the femur.

(5) Absence of pain.

(6) Absence of constitutional symptoms.

(7) Little or no spasm.

(8) Absence of shortening.

It is worthy of note that all these cases sought advice solely on account of the limp. It is also of interest that in two of the cases (the first and the fourth) the condition of flattening of the head of the femur exists on both sides; and it is of the greatest interest that in both cases there was entire absence of symptoms in one of the hips.

Direct injury, if severe enough, might cause a flattening of the head of the femur, and in children of this age the head is certainly impressionable. Should this be the cause in these cases, the thickening and shortening of the neck without evidence of fracture remains unexplained. We all know that the history of injury, especially in children, should be given much latitude, but in this group of cases, with a history of distinct injury in all of them, it seems to me that it must be considered, and at this time it seems to me that a possible explanation of the condition is that the injury may directly cause this condition by causing injury or displacement at the epiphyseal line, whereby the nutrition of the head, coming mostly through the neck, is impaired, and by the poorly nourished epiphysis bearing on the acetabulum, it becomes flattened. From such an injury a hyperemia of the neck of the femur would occur, and by this to stimulate bone growth the thickening of the neck may be explained.

Of the occurrence of a similar condition appearing in the apparently normal hip, I shall not, at this time, attempt to offer any explanation. Contre-coup and sympathetic inflammation may be considered, but these are, to my mind, very remote possibilities.

Apophysitis of the Tibial Tubercle

This seems to have been the only variety of osteochondritis that was appreciated before the era of X-ray diagnosis. In the last 30 years of the last century there were half a dozen accounts of this condition and that of Paget is included here. R. B. Osgood and C. Schlatter (1864-1935) independently described the X-ray appearances.

Periostosis Following Strains: Paget, 1891

... Much more common are the enlargements of the tubercle of the tibia which are often seen in young people much given to athletic games. They complain of aching pain at or about the part, especially during and after active exercise, and the tubercle may be felt enlarged, and is often too warm. The pain often continues more or less for many months, and there may be enlargement of the bursa under the ligamentum patellae, and the tubercle may remain too prominent; but common as are these cases, especially in our public schools, I have never known grave mischief ensue in any of them, and they get well of themselves. They may represent one of the least degrees of periostosis due to strain; the increase of the prominence of the bone is only just beyond that which may be deemed the normal limit for the attachment of vigorous muscles.

Robert Osgood, 1873-1956

Osgood had a great capacity for getting on well with people. After the First World War had brought English and American orthopaedic surgeons together, he encouraged this unity and assisted Robert Jones inaugurate the British Orthopaedic Association.

He was born in Salem, Massachusetts, and graduated from Harvard in 1899. At this time X-rays were the latest thing and as an intern at Massachusetts General Hospital Osgood helped the hospital pharmacist run the pioneer X-ray service. The following year he became Roentgenologist to the Boston Children's Hospital and wrote his first paper, on the disease which now bears his name. Fortunately his interest in radiology dwindled after this—the pharmacist subsequently developed X-ray cancers and eventually died, and Osgood himself developed many skin cancers but several operations prevented a fatal outcome.

After this paper he came to England to study, and worked with Robert Jones. He returned to Massachusetts General Hospital as an orthopaedic surgeon and studied the virology of polio amongst other things. With Goldthwait and Painter he wrote an orthopaedic textbook.

He suffered at one time from a tennis elbow. It did not improve with conservative measures so he was stimulated to think about its possible cause.

Thinking it might be due to a bursa lying between the muscles and the radio-humeral joint he went to the anatomy department where he found such a bursa in a cadaver. He had his own elbow explored under local anaesthetic and a bursa was excised. He never had any trouble again.

During the First World War he went to France with Harvey Cushing and later worked at Headquarters in London with Robert Jones who was directing the orthopaedic war effort.

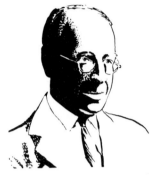

Lesions of the Tibial Tubercle Occurring during Adolescence:

by Robert B. Osgood, M.D., Boston   1903

(1) INTRODUCTION

Fractures of the tubercle of the tibia have for many years been recognised and have been considered almost as curiosities. The reported cases are nearly all those of fracture and marked separation, and are undoubtedly rare. There are, however, other lesions representing less severe forms of injury to the tubercle. These are interesting because they have apparently been seldom recognised and because of their comparatively frequent occurrence; because of the old difficulty of diagnosis and our present simple and accurate means, and because of their relation to the development of the tubercle.

(2) DEVELOPMENT OF THE TUBERCLE

The tubercle of the tibia develops ordinarily from the upper epiphysis of the tibia by the ossification of a tongue-like process extending downwards over the anterior surface of the diaphysis. Rarely there is a separate center of ossification for the tubercle which then develops as a separate epiphysis uniting with the upper epiphysis during the latter portion of adolescence.

(3) ANATOMY OF THE TUBERCLE DURING ADOLESCENCE

If in the light of development, the anatomy of the tubercle of the tibia in early adolescence is studied, it will be seen that the conditions are favorable for just the form of injuries to be described.

To the tip of a tongue-like process of bone, or to a separate bone center, is attached the tendon of one of the most powerful muscle groups in the body. This tongue or bone center is at the age at which the lesions occur separated from the strong shaft of bone by a layer of cartilage, and the first strain of the contraction of the quadriceps transmitted by the patella tendon comes on the tibial tubercle.

(4) REPORT OF DISSECTIONS AND EXPERIMENTS

Dissection—In a knee the skin and subcutaneous tissues were dissected back. The dissection was then carried upwards and the quadriceps muscle isolated. Traction upon this extended the knee, and the strain appeared to be taken first by the patella tendon, almost immediately followed by a tightening of these bands of accessory tendons.

With a chisel, the tibial tubercle was then fractured, leaving the patella tendon still attached to it. The few fibers of the tendon continued below the tubercle, and the slight insertion into the tendon of the above-mentioned lateral expansions were divided; the patella tendon was now isolated well above the deep bursa.

The conditions were now analogous to a complete fracture of the tubercle, and a detachment of the patella tendon from its point of pull.

The knee was flexed, and barely a quarter of an inch separation of the tubercle from its original situation occurred. The tubercle was then replaced and held loosely in position. By traction on the isolated quadriceps it was found that the knee could be practically fully extended without any difficulty, and that about one fourth of an inch displacement of the tubercle occurred. The first pull was transmitted mainly to the patella tendon and tubercle, and when that had yielded barely one fourth of an inch, it was adequately taken by the lateral expansions of the tendon of the quadriceps. The dissection made evident the strength of these expansions and their ability to act as tendons of insertion with a detached patella tendon, and also the fact that the knee could readily be extended with the attachment of the patella tendon gone.

(5) LESIONS OF THE TUBERCLE

We now come to lesions of the tubercle occurring during adolescence. These consist in a solution of continuity between the tubercle and the tibial shaft. They vary in severity from a complete avulsion of the tubercle to a slight separation of the epiphysis.

Separation of a fragment—It would seem from the experimental dissections that the first pull in a violent contraction of the quadriceps extensor comes on the fibres of the patella tendon, and is then taken also by the lateral expansions of the tendon of the quadriceps. In the complete avulsions and fractures, as stated above, we must suppose these accessory tendons to be torn from their attachments together with the tubercle and the patella tendon.

It is possible, however, to have a partial separation of the tubercle and the interference with normal function be so slight that the condition is often unrecognised and the diagnosis made of a bursitis or a periostitis, or even a joint fringe.

(1) *Clinical Picture.* These lesions occur in boys at or shortly after the age of puberty, when the epiphyseal growth is most rapid and a layer of cartilage intervenes between the epiphysis and the tibial shaft. In eight of the ten cases collected the boys were between fourteen and fifteen years of age; one was thirteen and the other sixteen. The boys were all active, athletic and well-developed muscularly. The histories and clinical pictures are very similar.

In the gymnasium, in running, in a football game, or in some athletic sport, the knee is "*strained*". This so-called strain is usually found on questioning to have been caused by the sudden violent extension of the leg; namely, by the strong contraction of the quadriceps. More rarely there is associated a fall on the flexed knee which would, of course, bring a sudden involuntary strain on the patella tendon, associated with trauma.

At the time of the injury there is felt acute pain in the knee referred to below the patella. There is often slight swelling, either general, or pretty definitely localised over the region of the tubercle. There is distinct tenderness at this point. The ability to use the leg is only slightly diminished, and the acute pain is soon replaced by a feeling of weakness on strong exertion. Sharp pain is present on violent extension or extreme flexion of the leg, and the patient usually consults the surgeon because of this pain, the annoying weakness and the continued localised swelling or tenderness.

The condition presents no complete loss of function, but a severe handicap to the active, athletic life which this class of patients wish to lead.

(2) *Diagnosis*—In these cases the thing clinically which we must suppose to occur, and which the x-rays confirm, is that a violent contraction or sudden strain of the quadriceps extensor partially ruptures the cartilaginous union of the tongue-like prolongation of the upper epiphysis or the separate ossifying center. A portion of this may be torn away, or perhaps the tongue may be simply separated to a variable extent.

Subsequent exertion of any kind, and sometimes the ordinary walking pull of the quadriceps, irritates the injured cartilage and gives rise to discomfort, until advice is sought or bony union at length takes place.

In two of the cases showing this lesion there had been no known wrench or trauma. The symptoms being the same as in the cases presenting recognised definite trauma.

(3) *Treatment*—The bursa directly above the tubercle and beneath the patella tendon in a small percentage of cases communicates directly with the joint. There may be enough bursitis set up to bring about a definite synovitis, for which complete immobilisation may be necessary. Ordinarily treatment directed toward lessening the pull of the patella tendon and restricting motion is adequate for the relief of the symptoms.

(4) *Prognosis*—The prognosis with treatment has been uniformly good as to relief of pain and restoration of function.

6 TRAUMA

Shock: Marshall Hall, 1790-1857

Marshall Hall was a son of the Industrial Revolution—the period when science came to the traditional arts. Hall, like Hunter, looked upon disease as an experiment devised by nature from which he could understand the physiology of the body. This is what clinical research meant to him.

He was born near Nottingham, where his father ran the family mill. His father discovered the bleaching action of chlorine and used it to bleach cotton; previously this had been achieved by leaving the cotton out in the sun for weeks. His brother remained in the business and made other innovations. Marshall Hall graduated from Edinburgh in 1812. In 1814 he made a tour of European centres and walked the 600 miles from Paris to Gottingen with a loaded pistol at the ready to fend off highwaymen and bandits.

On his return he set up as a physician in Nottingham at the age of 27, shortly afterwards publishing his first book *Diagnosis*, which was written whilst a student. The President of the Royal College of Physicians wrote to compliment him on this. On Hall's next visit to London he called upon the President. "I hope your father is well," said the President. "I, for one, am much indebted to him for his extraordinary work on *Diagnosis*." Dr. Hall modestly told him that he, not his father, was the author of the work. "Impossible," exclaimed the President, "it would have done credit to the greyest-headed philosopher in our profession." Whereupon he invited Dr. Hall to breakfast with him.

Hall was very struck by the frequence of death in labour associated with abdominal pain and bleeding. He described the features of shock which he observed in these patients and went on to question the value of therapeutic bleeding in a wide range of disorders. His paper produced a great change in the everyday practice of medicine; before it appeared venesection had been the universal remedy for any serious disease or accident. Hall's teaching that venesection was dangerous has perhaps prevented the loss of as many lives as more positive measures, such as the introduction of antibiotics, have saved.

In 1825, he was elected to the staff of the General Hospital, Nottingham; however, in the following year he took a trip to London, leaving no word about his return. After a while the Hospital authorities asked his relations when they were expecting him back. His brother-in-law wrote to him.

Marshall Hall told him to sell his house and all his belongings as he had decided to remain in London. He bought a house on a site now occupied by the Senate House of the University of London. He never had another hospital appointment. A steady stream of patients came to him as he acquired a name as a wise and kindly physician. "Our mission is to cure the curable," he wrote, "and comfort the incurable."

He married in 1829 and wrote a book on gynaecology. The following year he wrote an early infant welfare book, *Letters to a mother on the watchful care of her infant*.

At Nottingham he had observed disease and drawn far-reaching conclusions—in London, in a back room in Keppel Street, he began animal experimentation. He wrote about the circulation and was elected to the Royal Society in 1832. In the same year he read a paper before the Royal Society on spinal reflexes. The observation that a decapitated animal could still respond to stimuli led him to realise for the first time that the spinal cord, which had hitherto been looked upon as a cable joining the periphery with the brain, was itself capable of integrating sensory input and motor output. A second paper on the same subject the Royal Society refused to accept. He published it abroad and had nothing to do with the Royal Society again.

Marshall Hall was an intellectual Leviathan—he wrote about a decimal pharmacopoea, the emancipation of slaves, sewage plans for London, against flogging, and he introduced artificial respiration. He was a regular traveller, and went to the continent every year, frequently lecturing. In Italy he was often given the best rooms as his Christian name, Marshall, was thought to signify military rank. On the way to America, when everyone was sea-sick, he wrote a physiological paper on sea-sickness.

Paget found him "rather a sharp fellow" which perhaps explains why he followed such a solitary path and, like Hugh Owen Thomas, had no hospital appointment.

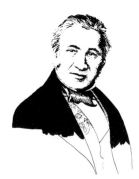

Marshall Hall: 1825

On Some Effects of Loss of Blood

The most familiar of the effects of loss of blood is Syncope. The influence of posture, and the first sensations and appearances of the patient, in this state, appear to denote that the brain is the organ the function of which is first impaired; the respiration suffers as an immediate consequence; and the action of the heart becomes enfeebled as an effect of the defect of stimulus—first from a deficient quantity of blood, and secondly from its deficient arterialisation; the capillary circulation also suffers; and if the state of syncope be long continued the stomach and the bowels become variously affected.

In ordinary syncope from loss of blood, the patient first experiences a degree of vertigo, to which loss of consciousness succeeds; the respiration is affected in proportion to the degree of insensibility—being suspended until the painful sensation produced rouses the patient to draw deep and repeated sighs, and again suspended as before; the beat of the heart and of the pulse is slow and weak; the face and general surface become pale, cool, and bedewed with perspiration; the stomach is apt to be effected with eructation or sickness. On recovery there is perhaps a momentary delirium, yawning, and a return of consciousness; irregular sighing breathing; and a gradual return of the pulse.

In cases of profuse haemorrhage the state of the patient varies:-there is at one moment a greater or lesser degree of syncope, then a degree of recovery. During the syncope the countenance is extremely pallid—there is more or less insensibility—the respiratory movements of the thorax are at one period imperceptible and then there are irregular sighs—the pulse is slow, feeble, or not to be distinguished—the extremities are apt to be cold, and the stomach is frequently affected with sickness. There are several phenomena observed in this state particularly worthy of attention. I have observed that when the movements of the chest have been imperceptible or nearly so, in the intervals between the sighs, the respiration has still been carried on by means of the *Diaphragm*. It may also be observed that the state of syncope is often relieved, for a time, by an attack of sickness and vomiting, immediately after which the patient expresses herself as feeling better, and the countenance is somewhat improved, the breathing more natural, and the pulse stronger and more frequent. It may be a question, in this case, whether the state of syncope increases until it induces sickness; or whether the stomach be nauseated by ingesta usually administered, and the syncope be, in part, an effect of this state of the stomach. In either case the efforts to vomit, are succeeded, for a time, by an amelioration in the state of the patient.

In cases of fatal haemorrhage there are none of these ameliorations. The symptoms gradually and progressively assume a more and more frightful aspect. The countenance does not improve but becomes more and more pale and shrunken; the consciousness sometimes remains until at the last there is some delirium; but everything denotes an impaired state of the brain; the breathing becomes stertorous and at length affected by a terrible gasping; there may be no attempt to vomit; the pulse is extremely feeble or even imperceptible; the animal heat fails and the extremities become colder and colder in spite of every kind of external warmth; the voice may be strong, and there are constant restlessness and jactitation; at length the strength fails, and the patient sinks, gasps and expires.

In 1830 in another article on this subject, he wrote:-

When Syncope assumes a dangerous form, the principal remedies are, an attention to the posture of the patient, stimulants, and chiefly brandy, and the transfusion of blood.

Rupture of the Tendo Achillis: Ambroise Paré (*Father of French Surgery*), 1510-1590

Ambroise Paré was born in Bourg Hersent in the old French province of Maine, where his father was a valet and barber. Several of his near relatives were in similar medical occupations. He studied with his brother Jean, and in 1532 was apprenticed to a Parisian barber-surgeon, then worked for four years at the Hôtel Dieu in Paris. He became a master barber-surgeon in 1541, and subsequently worked partly in Paris and partly as an army surgeon. He was surgeon to four Kings of France.

In 1575 he published a superb, monumental work on surgery. The first part is devoted to anatomy and physiology and the second to surgery, which includes descriptions of many surgical instruments; he re-introduced the ligation of vessels, and described prostheses for amputation.

He was one of the few Huguenots spared at the Massacre of St. Bartholomew.

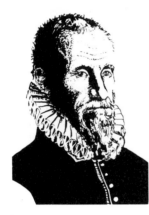

Paré: 1575

An Affect of the Large Tendon of the Heel

It oft times is rent or torn by a small occasion without any sign of injury or solution of continuity apparent on the outside as by a little jump, the slipping aside of the foot, the too nimble getting on horseback, or the slipping of the foot out of the stirrup in mounting into the saddle. When this chance happens, it will give a crack like a coachman's whip; above the head where the tendon is broken the depressed cavity may be felt with your finger; there is great pain in the part and the party is not able to go. This mischance may be amended by long lying and resting in bed and repelling medicines applied to the part . . . neither must we hereon promise to ourselves or the patient certain or absolute health. But on the contrary at the beginning of the disease we must foretell that it will never be so cured, and that some relics may remain. . . .

Pulled Elbow: Hugh Owen Thomas, 1834-1891

This short quick man, who was seen around the streets of Liverpool always wearing a black coat buttoned up to the neck, a second-mate's discharge cap, and a cigarette, came from a line of Anglesey bone-setters. His father was a successful bone-setter in Liverpool, and sent all his sons to Medical School. Hugh Owen qualified, and after a brief period working with his father, he became a general practitioner on his own. He never had a hospital appointment, and made a point of treating his patients at home. His special interests were lithopaxy, the management of the acute abdomen, and ortho-paedics. His ideas became accepted despite his unconventional background and his intolerance of others.

He was an advocate of enforced, prolonged and uninterrupted rest for the treatment of tuberculous joints. His armentarium of splints was superbly designed to achieve this and remain widely used: he devised the cervical collar, metatarsal bar, heel wedges, and the knee splint which is now called a Thomas splint. He was able to fit a patient at a few moments notice.

Robert Jones, his nephew, was brought up by Thomas and assisted him for a while; later Jones popularised his ideas and added his own, establishing the "Liverpool School" of Orthopaedics.

Thomas published a number of books written in a polemic style which give a good idea of his character and ideas.

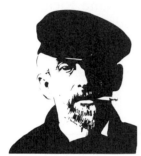

Pulled Elbow: Hugh Owen Thomas, 1883

This accident is invariably the result of applying traction and pronation by grasping the hand of the infant.

The mother or servant by whose agency the accident occurred, often brings the child for advice, and informs the surgeon that she only pulled him by the hand, which caused him to stumble whilst still held by the hand, and since then the arm had been disabled, and that the infant complained if any attempt were made to flex the elbow. On examination, the surgeon finds that the arm lies dependent, slightly flexed, and pronated, and that the child dreads being touched. If the arm be forcibly flexed and manipulated, it may or may not be instantly relieved—but this is not what the surgeon ought to do. There is a method which—if followed—is painless to the child, is immediately effectual, and favourably impresses any observers. We will here suppose that it is the right elbow. The surgeon must very gently grasp the child's hand with the thumb and index finger of his own right hand, planting his thumbs in the palmar base of the child's thumb while the index finger hooks round the ulnar edge and back of the child's hand, then placing the olecranon point of the child's elbow in the cupped palm of the surgeon's left hand, let him supinate the arm, and at the same time *fully* extend it, using the cupped palm of the left hand as a fulcrum; and now the surgeon in nearly every case will feel a click of some part slipping into place, and then let him instantly flex the elbow and fix in a sling.

The procedure is painless and the relief instant, and in nearly every case the little patient, after this operation, expresses a desire to use the elbow. Those in charge of the patient often imagine that the collar bone is the seat of the injury, the patient himself being too young to be interrogated, but the helpless, dependent and slightly flexed appearance of the arm, which is obvious at first sight, is always a safe guide. When operating on the left elbow, the surgeon must repeat the manipulation with the right hand behind the joint and the left in charge of the patient's hand.

Ischaemic Contracture: Richard von Volkmann, 1830-1889

The whole of Volkmann's life was spent in Halle, Saxony, where his father was Professor of Anatomy and Physiology. He studied at several universities and graduated at the age of 24. Two years later he became deputy Professor of Surgery and subsequently Director.

He instituted Lister's antiseptic methods at the hospital; it had previously been subject to so much infection that surgery was almost impossible.

He wrote poems and fairy stories with the pen name Richard Leander, which were very popular, and he also founded a surgical journal.

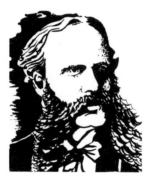

Ischaemic Muscular Paralyses and Contractures: Richard Volkmann, 1881

For many years I have been drawing attention to the fact that the paralyses and contractures of the limbs which sometimes follow bandages applied too tightly, do not arise, as was assumed, through paralysis of the nerves by pressure, but through wholesale and swift disintegration of the contractile substance and the resultant reaction and regeneration. The paralysis and contracture should be understood to have their origin in the muscle.

A series of new discoveries made since has established the correctness of this assertion, and at the same time has allowed us to obtain a more and more precise conception of the occurrences and processes in question. I should like to sum up here my present views as follows:

(1) The paralyses and contractures following tightly applied bandages, chiefly on the forearm and hand, and less often in the lower extremity, are to be viewed as ischaemic. They arise from the arterial blood supply being interrupted for too long. Venous stasis though occurring at the same time, does seem to accelerate the onset of the paralysis.

(2) The paralysis depends on the fact that the primary muscle groups die when deprived of oxygen for too long. The contractile substance coagulates, and disintegrates and becomes re-absorbed later. The resultant contracture is therefore most simply described as post-mortem stiffening; the paralysed and contracted limbs always show the same postures as we find in extremities in rigor mortis, if the total musculature of a limb or part of a limb is simultaneously affected.

(3) It is a feature that paralysis and contracture always appear simultaneously or follow each other closely, whilst in nervous paralysis of the extremities the contracture always develops very gradually and often very late. In the latter cases months and years may elapse before a deformity develops which can no longer be overcome by strong manual force.

(4) By contrast from the first moment of the appearance of an ischaemic contracture there is tremendous resistance to correction of the deformity. The affected muscles completely lose their elasticity and are absolutely rigid at an early stage, so resembling rigor mortis.

(5) Necrosis of the contractile substance is followed by reactive and regenerative processes of which the latter always remains very incomplete in man; the affected muscles become more unyielding and the contracture increased still further by cicatricial shrinkage.

(6) Ischaemic paralysis and contractures of identical nature appear not only after the application of unduly tight bandages and the unduly prolonged Esmarch's constriction of the limbs, but also after ligatures, avulsions and contusions of large vessels, but perhaps too after the prolonged exposure to cold. It is possible that some of the so-called rheumatic contractures are of an ischaemic nature.

(7) Kraske has clearly shewn in his beautiful work that animal muscle cannot withstand the complete occlusion of the arterial blood supply for six hours without a great number of fibres perishing, and that after six hours of complete deprivation the most violent reactionary processes develop, which is a reminder of the so-called auto-digestion. The fact that there have been no unfavourable experiences up till now so far as I know although the rubber bandages are often left in position for hours at a time, does not count for much, because the great majority of these patients have certainly perished. After the application of tight bandages, however, the ischaemia will almost never be complete. The degree of severity of the sequelae will depend upon the completeness of the ischaemia, and whether many or few fibres were affected by it. If the ischaemia is very considerable such alarming phenomena appear so quickly that the bandage will be removed; even so, half a day and less is enough to reduce the fingers to permanent and pitiful deformity. If the constriction is less marked and the bandage left in place for a week in spite of complaints of pain, in spite of oedema and cyanosis of fingers and toes, the result is still only a moderate contracture and a moderate loss of muscle fibre. In particular such moderate contractures are frequently observed after Fractura Radii Typica. The residual slight flexion of the fingers yields here, too, only after many months of continuous and energetic treatment.

(8) The prognosis of ischaemic muscle paralysis and contracture will therefore depend upon the number of fibres which have necrosed or disintegrated. The severest cases affecting the hand and fingers are to be considered absolutely incurable. The prognosis is better in the lower extremity, because here the main symptom, i.e. muscular

shortening, can easily be removed by tenotomy. The milder cases are improved and cured only by the most energetic and consistent treatment.

(9) Anything other than mechanical aids will prove completely useless. For very recent ischaemic contractures one should try to stretch the shortened and stiff muscles by the application of force under chloroform anaesthesia before anything else. In all older cases this is unsuccessful; one would more readily break the bones and rupture the tendons before the muscles would yield.

FRACTURES

The surgeon ought to be very cautious in delivering his prognostic concerning fractures. He should avoid being too hasty in promising a quick, easy, and certain cure, lest his art should be overcome by accidental disorders, and he should be accused of Knavery or Ignorance.

Heister, 1683-1758.

Colles' Fracture: Abraham Colles, 1773-1843

Colles was born near Kilkenny, Ireland. The story goes that while he was at school, a flood swept through the local doctor's house, carrying away his possessions. One of his anatomy books landed up near the Colles' home. Abraham found it, and on returning it to the doctor, he was made a present of the book. This is thought to have turned his mind towards medicine.

He trained at Dublin and then went to Edinburgh for post-graduate study. After obtaining the degree of M.D. in 1797, he walked from Edinburgh to London. The following year he settled in surgical practice in Dublin, and was elected President of the Royal College of Surgeons of Ireland at the age of 29. He wrote a book on surgical anatomy in 1811 and a paper on club foot in 1818. His paper on radial fractures was published in 1814, followed in 1837 by a book on venereal disease and the use of mercury. An early riser, he ran one of the most lucrative practices in Dublin.

"As an operator he has many equals, and some superiors; but in advice, from long experience and a peculiar tact in discovering the hidden causes of disease, he has scarcely a rival." So wrote a contemporary.

On Fracture of the Carpal Extremity of the Radius: Abraham Colles, 1814

The injury to which I wish to direct the attention of surgeons has not, as far as I know, been described by any other author; indeed

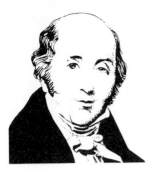

the form of the carpal extremity would rather induce us to question its being liable to fracture. The absence of crepitus, and of the other common symptoms of fracture, together with the swelling which instantly arises in this, as in other injuries of the wrist, render the difficulty of ascertaining the real nature of the case very considerable.

This fracture takes place about an inch and a half above the carpal extremity of the radius, and exhibits the following appearances :-

The posterior surface of the limb presents a considerable deformity; for a depression is seen in the fore-arm, about an inch and a half above the end of this bone, while a considerable swelling occupies the wrist and metacarpus. Indeed the carpus and base of the metacarpus appear to be thrown backwards so much as on first view to excite a suspicion that the carpus had been dislocated forward.

On observing the anterior surface of the limb, we observe a considerable fullness, as if caused by the flexor tendons being thrown forwards. This fullness extends upwards to about one third of the length of the fore-arm, and terminates below at the upper edge of the annular ligament of the wrist. The extremity of the ulna is seen projecting towards the palm and inner edge of the limb; the degree, however, in which this projection takes is different in different instances.

If the surgeon proceeds to investigate the nature of this injury he will find that the end of the ulna admits of being readily moved backwards and forwards.

On the posterior surface he will discover, by the touch, that the swelling on the wrist and metacarpus is not caused entirely by the effusion among the soft parts; he will perceive that the ends of the metacarpal and second row of carpal bones form no small part of it. This, strengthening the suspicion which the first view of the case had excited, leads him to examine, in a more particular manner, the anterior part of the joint; but the want of that solid resistance which a dislocation of the carpus forwards must occasion forces him to abandon this notion, and leaves him in a state of perplexing uncertainty as to the real nature of the injury. He will, therefore, endeavour to gain some information by examining the bones of the forearm. The facility with which (as was noticed) the ulna can be moved backward and forward does not furnish him with any useful hint. When he moves his fingers along the anterior surface of the radius he finds it more full and prominent than is natural; a similar examination of the posterior surface of this bone induces him to think that a depression is felt about an inch and a half above its carpal extremity. He now expects to find satisfactory proofs of a fracture of the radius at this spot. For this purpose he attempts to move the broken pieces of bone in opposite directions; but, although the patient is by this examination excited by considerable pain, yet neither crepitus nor a yielding of the bone at the seat of the fracture, nor any other positive evidence of the existence of such an injury, is thereby obtained. The patient complains of severe pain as often as an attempt is made to give to the limb the motions of pronation and supination.

If the surgeon lock his hand in that of the patient and make extension, even with considerable force, he restores the limb to its natural form, but the distortion of the limb instantly returns on the extension being removed. Should the facility with which a moderate extension restores the limb to its form induce the practitioner to treat this as a case of sprain, he will find, after a lapse of time sufficient for the removal of similar swellings, the deformity undiminished. Or, should he mistake the case for a dislocation of the wrist, and attempt to retain the parts in situ by tight bandages and splints, the pain caused by the pressure on the back of the wrist will force him to unbind them in a few hours; and if they be applied more loosely, he will find, at the expiration of a few weeks, that the deformity still exhibits in its fullest extent, and that it is now no longer to be removed by making extension of the limb. By such mistakes the patient is doomed to endure for many months considerable lameness and stiffness of the limb, accompanied by severe pains on attempting to bend the hand and fingers. One consolation only remains, that the limb at some remote period will again enjoy perfect freedom in all its motions, and be completely exempt from pain; the deformity, however, will remain undiminished throughout life.

The unfavourable result of some of the first cases of this description which came under my care forced me to investigate with peculiar anxiety the nature of the injury. But while the absence of crepitus and of the other usual symptoms of fracture render the diagnosis extremely difficult, a recollection of the superior strength and thickness of this part of the radius, joined to the mobility of its articulation with the carpus and ulna, rather inclined me to question the possibility of a fracture taking place at this part of the bone. At last, after many unsuccessful trials, I hit upon the following simple method of examination by which I was enabled to ascertain that the symptoms above enumerated actually rose from a fracture seated about one and half inches above the carpal extremity of the radius.

Let the surgeon apply the fingers of one hand to the seat of the suspected fracture, and, locking the other hand in that of the patient, make a moderate extension until he observes the limb restored to its natural form. As soon as this is effected let him move the patients hand backward and forward, and he will, at every such attempt, be sensible of yielding of the fractured ends of the bone, and this to such a degree as must remove all doubt from his mind.

The nature of this injury, once ascertained, will be a very easy matter to explain, the different phenomena attendant on it, and to point out a method of treatment which will prove completely successful. The hard swelling which appears on the back of the hand is caused by the carpal surface of the radius being directed slightly backwards instead of looking directly downwards. The carpus and metacarpus, retaining their connections with this bone, must follow it in its derangements and cause the convexity above alluded to. This change of direction in the articulating surface of the radius is caused by the tendons of the exterior surface of the thumb, which pass along the posterior surface of the radius in sheaths firmly connected with the inferior extremity of this bone. The broken extremity of the radius being thus drawn backwards causes the ulna to appear prominent towards the palmar surface, while it is probably thrown more towards the inner or ulnar side of the limb by the upper end of the fragment of the radius pressing against it in that direction. The separation of these two bones from each other is facilitated by a previous rupture of their capsular ligament, an event which may be readily occasioned by the violence of the injury. An effusion in the sheaths of the flexor tendons will account for that swelling which occupies the limb anteriorly.

It is obvious that in the treatment of this fracture our attention should be principally directed to guard against the carpal end of the radius being drawn backwards. For this purpose, while assistants hold the limb in a middle state between pronation and supination, let a thick and firm compress be applied transversely on the anterior surface of the limb, at the seat of the fracture, taking care that it shall not press on the ulna; let this be bound on firmly with a roller and then let a tin splint, formed to the shape of the arm, be applied to both its anterior and posterior surfaces. In cases where the end of the ulna is much displaced, I have laid a very narrow wooden splint along the naked side of the bone. This latter splint, I now think, should be used in every instance, as, by pressing the extremity of the ulna against the side of the radius, it will tend to oppose the displacement of the fractured end of this bone. It is scarcely necessary to observe that the two principal splints should be much more narrow at the wrist than those in general use, and should also extend to the roots of the fingers, spreading out so as to give a firm support to the hand. The cases treated on this plan have all recovered without the smallest defect or deformity of the limb, in the ordinary time for the care of fractures.

I cannot conclude these observations without remarking that were my opinion to be drawn from those cases only which have occurred to me, I should consider this as by far the most common injury to which the wrist or carpal extremities are exposed. During the last three years I have not met a single instance of Desault's dislocation of the inferior end of the radius, while I have had opportunities of seeing a vast number of the fracture of the lower end of this bone.

Smith's Fracture: Robert William Smith

*Fracture of the Lower Extremity of the Radius, with
Displacement of the Lower Fragment Forwards*
1847

This is an injury of exceedingly rare occurrence, and one which presents characters closely resembling those of dislocation of the carpus forwards. It generally occurs in consequence of a fall upon the back of the hand, and the situation of the fracture is from half an inch to an inch above the articulation; it is accompanied by great deformity, the principal features of which are a dorsal and a palmar tumour, and a striking projection of the head of the ulna at the posterior and inner part of the fore-arm; the dorsal tumour occupies the entire breadth of the fore-arm; but is most conspicuous internally, where it is constituted by the lower extremity of the ulna displaced backwards; from this point, the inferior outline of the tumour passes obliquely upwards and outwards, corresponding in the latter direction to the lower end of the superior fragment of the radius. Immediately below the dorsal swelling there is a well-marked sulcus, deepest internally below the head of the ulna, directed nearly transversely, but ascending a little as it approaches the radial border of the fore-arm.

The palmar is less remarkable than the dorsal tumour; formed principally by the lower fragment of the radius, it is obscured by the thick mass of flexor tendons which cross the front of the carpus, but towards the ulnar border of the limb there is a considerable projection, which marks the situation of the pisiform bone, passing down to its attachment into which, can be seen the tendon of the flexor carpi ulnaris thrown forwards in strong relief. The transverse diameter of the fore-arm is not much altered, but the antero-posterior is considerably increased, and the radial border of the limb becomes concave at its lowest part.

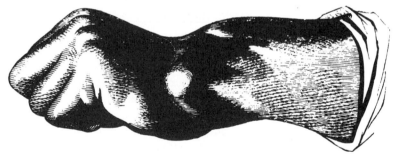

Smith's Fracture

In the case from which the preceding drawings was made, the patient, in endeavouring to save himself from being run over by a car, fell with great violence upon the back of his hand; the lower end of the radius was broken and driven forwards along with the carpus, and the head of the ulna was displaced backwards.

I cannot speak with accuracy as to the anatomical characters of the injury, having never had an opportunity of examining after death the skeleton of the fore-arm, in those who had during life met with this accident; nor is there any preparation shewing the exact relative position of the fragments, in any of the pathological collections in Dublin; but still I feel satisfied that the injury, the external characters of which have just been described, is a feature of the lower end of the radius, with displacement of the lower fragment along the carpus forwards, and of the head of the ulna backwards, and that it has not unfrequently been mistaken for dislocation of the carpus forwards and of the bones of the fore-arm backwards.

The facility, however, with which the deformity can be removed, its liability to recur when the extending force ceases to act, the production of crepitus when the limb is extended, and a motion of rotation given to the hand, and our being able to feel the irregular margin of the upper fragment of the radius posteriorly, are sufficient to enable us to distinguish this accident from luxation of the bones of the wrist forwards.

Bennett's Fracture: Edward Hallaran Bennett, 1837-1907

The son of the Recorder of Cork, Bennett studied at Trinity College, Dublin. Soon after qualifying he established himself as an anatomist at the University and built up a wonderful collection of specimens of bone pathology, and he drew on this to write his papers on metacarpal fractures in which he mentioned the fracture dislocation of the thumb which bears his name.

In 1873 he succeeded Smith as Professor of Surgery at Trinity College, Dublin. He was a stimulating teacher, the model of honour and uprightness, who never did a crooked thing, and was blunt but not unkind. He became President of the Royal College of Surgeons of Ireland.

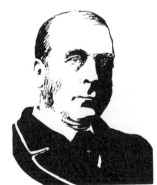

Fractures of the Metacarpal Bones: E. H. Bennett, 1882

The specimens I submit are united fractures of the third and fifth metacarpals of the same right hand, one of the shaft and one of the base of the fifth, both from right hands, and five of the first, all from the right side.

These are the entire number of these fractures which I have collected, and most remarkable is the fact that they are all of the right side. They show, so far as their evidence is of value, that the bones most frequently the subject of fracture are the first and fifth metacarpals of the right side.

Of greater interest is the fact that in each of the five examples of fracture of the metacarpal bone of the thumb, allowing for shades of difference such as must always exist, the type and character of the fracture is the same—a form and type of fracture not hitherto described in these bones; and if this series be of any value as representing the ordinary injuries, the commonest fracture, certainly the most common of thumb, possibly of all the bones taken together, is that the characters of which are seen in this specimen, in which least of all have the lines of fracture been marked by changes on the articular surface which corresponds to trapezium. The fracture passes obliquely (*a b* in woodcut) through the base of the bone, detaching the greater part of the articular facette with that piece of bone supporting it, which projects into the palm. The amount of displacement in this and all the specimens is trivial, and from clinical observation of the injury it is evident that the fragment displaced is not the smaller, as one might infer from an examination of the

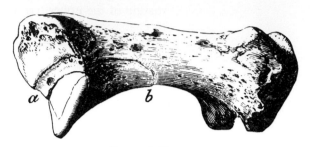

Bennett's Fracture

isolated specimens of united fractures, but the larger—in fact, to the extent that the irregularity of the surface indicates that the metacarpal bone of the thumb undergoes subluxation backwards. In all these specimens the dorsal surface of the bone is free from any implication in the fracture, and this fact, combined with the small amount of displacement which occurs, renders the fracture one extremely liable to escape detection. The importance of a correct diagnosis of this injury is illustrated by a case which I have had for nearly two years under observation. A girl, aged twenty, was thrown from an outside car and fell to the ground, saving herself from graver injury by putting forward her arm; she struck the ball of the thumb against the ground; and at once suffered extreme pain in it. Next morning I saw her at Sir P. Dun's Hospital, when at first sight no injury was apparent beyond the swelling of a bruised and sprained thumb. In handling the ball of the thumb I felt osseus crepitus, and, having my attention so arrested, I was not long in establishing the diagnosis of this injury, for the dorsal surface of the metacarpal was entire; it projected backwards at the articulation with the carpus, and by reducing it into place crepitus could easily be elicited. So trivial an injury does this appear to be, and the specimens show so little deformity, except in some the sign of arthritis consequent on it, I might fairly be asked what importance attaches to the correct diagnosis. All will admit that a correct diagnosis even in trivial injuries is desirable, but in this case the diagnosis is essential to a correct prognosis, and here lies the importance of the injury. Seeing the value of the movement of the thumb, no injury of it is to be lightly regarded, and this fracture, though it unites readily by bone and with almost inappreciable deformity, renders the thumb for many months lame and useless. In the case I have reported, even now, nearly two years after the accident occurring in a young and healthy subject, the hand fails to grasp or lift with certainty any body requiring a wide gape of the thumb—for instance, to lift a tumbler full of water from the table, and this in a case where every care was taken to keep the parts in place and at rest for a proper time.

Monteggia's Fracture: Giovanni Battista Monteggia, 1762-1815

Monteggia was born at Lake Maggiore and studied at Milan. At first he was a surgical pathologist; whilst performing an autopsy on a woman who had died of syphilis he had the misfortune to cut his finger and infected himself with the disease. Later he became a successful general surgeon and pleased one patient so much that he was given an annuity to keep his library up-to-date.

When he became Professor of Surgery at Milan he published his lectures which are remarkable for the wide acquaintance with the work of his contemporaries. He is particularly remembered for his description of a fracture dislocation of the forearm which he described in the same year as Colles described his fracture.

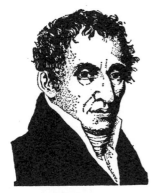

Monteggia's Fracture: 1814

I unhappily remember the case of a girl who, after a fall, seemed to me to have sustained a fracture of the ulna in its upper third. It might have been that some commotion of the dislocated bone misled me at the beginning of treatment, or else it might have been that there really was a fracture of the ulna with a dislocation of the radius, as I undoubtedly found in another case. The fact is that at the end of the month, when the bandage was removed and all the swelling had disappeared (which, however, in simple dislocation of the radius is usually slight), I found that on extending the forearm the head of the radius jumped outwards, forming a hard ugly prominence on the anterior surface of the elbow, showing in an extremely obvious way that this was a true anterior dislocation of the head of the radius. When compressed it went back into place, but left to itself it came out again especially on extension of the forearm. I applied compresses and a new bandage to hold it in, but it would not stay in place.

Galeazzi's Fracture: Riccardo Galeazzi, 1866-1952

Fractures of the forearm should be superbly treated in Milan; Monteggia was there and then Galeazzi, who between them described upper and lower dislocations which may accompany fractures of one bone only.

Galeazzi was director of the orthopaedic clinic for 35 years; he built up the unit and established ancillary centres. He was a prolific writer on many topics—for example, he reviewed 12,000 cases of congenital dislocation of the hip.

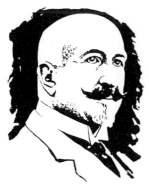

Concerning a Particular Syndrome of Injury of the Forearm Bones: R. Galeazzi, 1934

We have observed, with relative frequency, a fracture of the diaphysis of the radius at the junction of the middle and lower thirds combined with luxation of the ulnar head. In this form of trauma we have a repetition of the Monteggia syndrome: i.e. one bone remains uninjured while the other is fractured.

The consequent shortening of the radius is probably one of the important causes of the subluxation or dislocation of the distal radio-ulnar joint, as occurs in the proximal joint in fractures of the ulna.

The angulation of the radial fracture is sometimes lateral and sometimes posterior; and the luxation of the ulnar head may be anterior, dorsal or medial, all with more or less equal frequency though medial displacement is perhaps most common. Fracture of the ulnar styloid with displacement of the distal fragment towards the radius is fairly common.

As for the relative incidence of the present syndrome and that of Monteggia—my material shows that the distal syndrome is much more common: in 300 cases of forearm fractures that I have collected, the Monteggia injury accounted for 2% of the cases, whereas the injury that I am describing accounted for 6%.

Both the proximal and distal syndromes may follow direct or indirect injuries. I, myself, have encountered more cases of the present syndrome than that of Monteggia, arising from indirect injury, such as a fall on the palm of the hand with the arm abducted.

Galeazzi then describes with great formality and at considerable length the mechanical forces responsible for the two injuries. He points out that the axis of the forearm passes through the humero-ulnar joint at the upper end and through the radio-carpal joint at the lower end. Both these joints are formed by the strongest ends of the bones. The other ends of the bones are weakly linked to the humerus above and to the carpus below. In a fall on the hand the compression force on the forearm bones may cause a fracture of one of them at the point of maximal bowing, for example at the junction of the middle and the lower third of the radius. If the force continues to operate, either the ulnar will fracture or the distal arm will pivot at the fracture site, putting a strain on the inferior radio-ulnar ligament. If this ruptures, dislocation of the head of the ulna follows.

When the fracture is due to direct violence then muscle shortening produces overlapping. Again the distal arm pivots and the ligament may rupture.

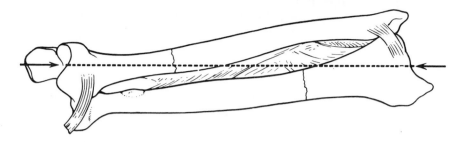

Galeazzi compares the injury that he described with that described by Monteggi.

Galeazzi mentions that the dislocation may develop slowly during the course of treatment for what initially appears to be a solitary fracture.

He discusses treatment and we return to his words for an account of this.

> In my experience traction has always yielded the best results. The distal fragment of the radius is usually pronated by pronator quadratus and displaced towards the ulna by abductor pollicis bowstringing across it.
>
> In my experience, energetic traction on the thumb with the hand in supination has always permitted immediate reduction of the fracture, then by deviating the hand radially the dislocated ulnar head is reduced without further manipulation. Only if the diastasis of the inferior radio-ulnar joint is very severe, because the ligaments have suffered total rupture, does the dislocation tend to recur; it is then necessary to transfix both bones with threads after reduction.

Pott's Fracture: Percivall Pott, 1714-1788

Some years after Pott had suffered a compound fracture of the tibia, he wrote this account. Judging from his son-in-law's description of the injury, which appears on page 7, it is unlikely that he suffered the fracture that bears his name.

Remarks on Fractures and Dislocations: 1769

There is a case which, according to the general manner of treating it, gives infinite pain and trouble both to the patient and surgeon, and very frequently ends in the lameness and disappointment of the former, and the disgrace and concern of the latter—I mean the fracture of the fibula attended with a dislocation of the tibia.

Whoever will take a view of the leg of a skeleton, will see that although the fibula be a very small and slender bone, and very inconsiderable in strength, when compared with the tibia, yet the support of the lower joint of that limb (the ancle), depends so much on this slender bone, that without it the body would not be upheld, nor locomotion performed, without hazard of dislocation every moment. The lower extremity of this bone, which descends considerably below the end of the tibia, is by strong and inelastic ligaments firmly connected with the last-named bone, and with the astragalus, or that bone of the tarsus which is principally concerned in forming the joint of the ancle. This lower extremity of the fibula has, in its posterior part, a superficial sulcus for the lodgment and passage of the tendons of the peronei muscles, which are here tied down by strong ligamentous capsulae, and have their action so determined from this point or angle, that the smallest degree of variation from it, in consequence of external force, must necessarily have considerable effect on the motions they are designed to execute, and consequently distort the foot. Let it also be considered, that upon the due and natural state of the joint of the ancle, that is, upon the exact and proper disposition of the tibia and fibula, both with regard to each other and to the astragalus, depend the just disposition and proper action of several other muscles of the foot and toes; such as the gastrocnemii, the tibialis anticus and posticus, the flexor pollicis longus, and the flexor digitorum pedis longus, as must appear demonstrably to any man who will first dissect, and then attentively consider these parts.

If the tibia and fibula be both broken, they are both generally displaced in such manner, that the inferior extremity, or that connected with the foot, is drawn under that part of the fractured bone which is connected with the knee; making by this means a deformed, unequal tumefaction in the fractured part, and rendering the broken limb shorter than it ought to be, or than its fellow. And this is generally the case, let the fracture be in what part of the leg it may.

If the tibia only be broken, and no act of violence, indiscretion, or inadvertence be committed, either on the part of the patient or of those who conduct him, the limb most commonly preserves its figure and length; the same thing generally happens if the fibula only be broken, in all that part of it which is superior to letter A in the annexed figure, or in any part of it between its upper extremity, and within two or three inches of its lower one.

I have already said, and it will obviously appear to every one who examines it, that the support of the body, and the due and proper use and execution of the office of the joint of the ancle, depend almost entirely on the perpendicular bearing of the tibia upon the astragalus, and on its firm connexion with the fibula. If either of these be perverted or prevented, so that the former bone is forced from its just and perpendicular position on the astragalus; or if it be separated by violence from its connexion with the latter, the joint of the ancle will suffer a partial dislocation internally; which partial dislocation cannot happen without not only a considerable extension, or perhaps laceration of the bursal ligament of the joint, which is lax and weak, but a laceration of those strong tendinous ligaments, which connect the lower end of the tibia with the astragalus and os calcis, and which constitute in great measure the ligamentous strength of the joint of the ancle.

This is the case, when, by leaping or jumping, the fibula breaks in the weak part already mentioned; that is, within two or three inches of its lower extremity. When this happens, the inferior fractured end of the fibula falls inward toward the tibia, that extremity of the bone which forms the outer ancle is turned somewhat outward and upward, and the tibia having lost its proper support, and not being of itself capable of steadily preserving its true perpendicular bearing, is forced off from the astragalus inwards, by which means

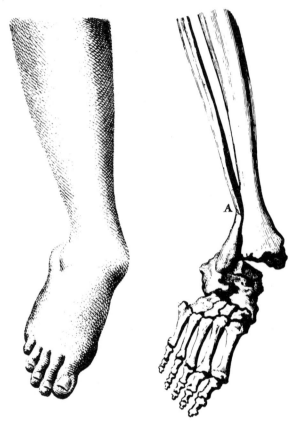

Pott's Fracture

the weak bursal, or common ligament of the joint, is violently stretched, if not torn, and the strong ones, which fasten the tibia to the astragalus and os calcis, are always lacerated; thus producing at the same time a perfect fracture and partial dislocation, to which is sometimes added a wound in the integuments, made by the bone at the inner ancle. By this means and indeed as a necessary consequence, all the tendons which pass behind or under, or are attached to the extremities of the tibia and fibula, or os calcis, have their natural direction and disposition so altered, that instead of performing their appointed actions, they all contribute to the distortion of the foot, and that by turning it outward and upward.

When this accident is accompanied, as it sometimes is, with a wound of the integuments of the inner ancle, and that made by the protrusion of the bone, it not infrequently ends in a fatal gangrene, unless prevented by timely amputation, though I have several times seen it do very well without. But in its most simple state, unaccompanied with any wound, it is extremely troublesome to put to rights, still more so to keep it in order, and unless managed with address and skill, is very frequently productive both of lameness and deformity ever after.

Dupuytren's Fracture: 1819

Baron Dupuytren gave a lecture on fractures and dislocations of the ankle, describing the varieties that he had observed, and, in an appendix, provided a statistical analysis of their frequency and outcome.

Dupuytren's Fracture

Dislocation of the foot outwards and upwards.—This form of displacement is so rare that I have only seen it once in nearly two hundred cases of fractured fibula which have fallen under my observation in the last fifteen years. It involves not only fracture of the fibula, but also laceration of the strong tibio-peroneal ligaments, which generally resist a force to which the osseous tissue itself yields. The following is the remarkable case to which I refer.

Case XVI. *Fracture of the fibula and rupture of ligaments, with dislocation of the foot upwards and outwards.* C. N. Guillemain, a joiner, aged 54, of sanguine temperament, was coming half-drunk out of a pot-house, for the purpose of making water, when, reeling along in a hurried manner, he came to an inclined and slippery piece of ground, where he fell, his right leg being extended outwards from the body, the weight of which it had to sustain together with the superadded momentum of the fall. Being unable to walk, he was immediately conveyed to the Hôtel-Dieu. This occurred in the winter of 1816.

When admitted, the presence of the usual signs indicating fractured fibula low down were readily detected; but what most attracted attention was the shortness of the leg, together with the almost doubled interval comprised between the maleoli, and the prolongation of the tibia downwards to a level with the sole of the foot: the astragalus and outer malleolus, with the whole of the foot, were drawn up on the outer side of the tibia, two inches above their normal position. All these signs left no doubt that the ligaments connecting the tibia and fibula were torn through, and that the foot was dislocated outwards and upwards, carrying with it the outer malleolus.

The swelling, tension, and pain momentarily increasing, it was necessary at once to reduce the parts; and this was satisfactorily accomplished after the patient had been bled. The foot and leg then resumed their natural form and direction and my apparatus for fractured fibula was forthwith applied, and an evaporating lotion laid over the joint.

On the following day the apparatus was removed with a view to re-apply it, and in consequence of an involuntary contraction of the muscles, the parts were again thrown out of place: the reduction was more readily affected this time by distracting the attention of the patient, and the apparatus was again adjusted: a second bleeding was ordered, and low diet prescribed.

On the third day the tension, swelling, and pain had nearly subsided; and from this time, strange to say, considering the serious mischief which must have existed, the case proceeded as if it had been one of simple fracture; so that on the thirty-sixth day the patient began to walk with crutches, and there was not the slightest irregularity in the form of the injured limb. He speedily regained his strength; and when seen six months afterwards, he retained only the recollection of the accident, without any of the consequences which it originally threatened.

Freiberg's Infraction: Albert H. Freiberg, 1868-1940

Freiberg spent all his life in his birthplace, Cincinnati, apart from a period of study in Germany and Austria. He established himself as an orthopaedic surgeon in the city and played an important part in the establishment of orthopaedic facilities there. His influence on the development of American orthopaedics was felt for two reasons: first, he was an active medical author, one of the leaders of thought—he has been called the philosopher of orthopaedic surgery. The second reason for his eminence was his committee-manship; an able, kindly speaker, he had the ability to turn discussions.

He is best remembered for describing flattening of the head of the second metatarsal. It is interesting to note that he considered that it was an injury. Since then opinion has swung towards osteochondritis and back again; most people would now agree that Freiberg was right.

In 1910-11 he was President of the American Orthopaedic Association. It is ironic that Freiberg, whose name is attached to the second metatarsal, should have just missed working with Keller, who campaigned against damaging the first metatarsal head, at the Walter Reed Hospital. Freiberg spent the war there and Keller joined the staff after it was over.

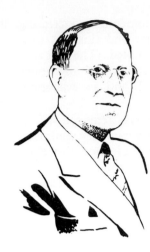

Infraction of the Second Metatarsal Bone

A TYPICAL INJURY

by Albert H. Freiberg, M.D., F.A.C.S., Cincinnati, Ohio, 1914

As a part of the general symptom-complex of weak or so-called "flat foot" we very commonly encounter pain in the forefoot, in the region of the metatarsal heads. When seen as a paroxysmal affection concerning the fourth metatarsal, in particular, we are dealing with the metatarsalgia of Morton. Very frequently, however, we are consulted by patients because of pain in the heads of the other metatarsals which is not of paroxysmal character but rather dependent upon the use of the foot in weight-bearing. This may or may not be in the presence of other signs of yielding and strain in the foot mechanism elsewhere than in the metatarsal region, but the dependence of the pain purely upon the weight-bearing function will cause us to ascribe the symptom to static incompetence of the foot. Under these circumstances we shall find that the most common seat of the pain is the second metatarso-phalangeal joint instead of the fourth, as in Morton's disease. The joint is usually tender to pressure and frequently somewhat thickened. The well-known plantar callus is frequently seen; almost uniformly so in cases of long standing. I have often found thickening of such degree in the second metatarso-phalangeal joint that I have sought for organic change in the radiogram; always without finding it, however, until I encountered Case 1 of the series which I am now reporting. In this case I felt justified in the diagnosis of infraction of the distal end of the second metatarsal, a condition which I have thus far failed to find described in literature.

During the past few years I have encountered six cases of infraction of the distal end of the second metatarsal bone. I feel justified in speaking of it as a typical injury because in each of my six cases not only was the same bone end involved, but the conditions under which the patients presented themselves were very similar, as was also the character of the trauma which produced the lesion.

Ten years ago the first patient in whom I recognised this lesion was referred to me by Dr. E. W. Mitchell, of Cincinnati. The patient was a girl of sixteen. She had been suffering from pain in the ball of the foot for about six months. The pain was precisely like that which we so often encounter in the metatarso-phalangeal region in connection with static incompetence of the foot. At the time I examined the patient she complained of pain in weight-bearing only. In attempting any unusual exertion, as in walking considerable distances, she was compelled to limp and the pain became severe.

The patient was quite sure that the condition dated from and was due to a game of tennis in which she "stubbed" her foot. The pain was severe at the time; it was considered a sprain and she was able to be about the next day.

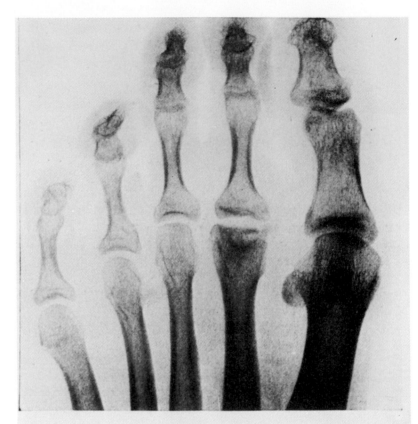

Fig. 1. Case 1. Girl of sixteen years. Tennis injury six months before. Infraction of second metatarsal with one small loose body. No arthrotomy required.

Frieberg's Infraction

My examination disclosed a well formed and apparently strong foot. The metatarsophalangeal articulation of the second toe was thickened, on palpation, and very tender to pressure. Passive movement of this joint was very painful and accomplished by slight grating. The X-ray (Fig. 1) showed quite clearly that the distal end of the second metatarsal had been crushed in, causing the articular surface to lose its curved outline. There was apparently a small loose body in the joint about two mm. in diameter.

The treatment consisted in applying a felt pad to the plantar surface of the foot by means of adhesive plaster, so that its anterior end was placed just back of the injured joint. In this case I also had a steel plate inserted between the layers of the sole of the boot in order to deprive the foot of the motion in the metatarsophalangeal joints, in walking. I have not done this in my later cases.

The patient was able to walk painlessly without the pad within six weeks and has had no further trouble with this foot. The other foot has always been entirely normal.

I find it unnecessary to report each of my cases in detail, as they have great similarity except as noted below.

Three of my six cases have shown loose bodies in the radiogram, and grating upon examination. In two of these three cases I was unable to give definite relief by mechanical support alone and, therefore, removed the loose bodies by means of an arthrotomy from the dorsal surface of the foot. This resulted in entire relief from discomfort and pain.

It is a curious fact that in two of the six cases, no injury whatever could be recalled by the patients in spite of careful questioning on my part. In one of these cases operative removal of small corpora libera was necessary. I have no doubt of the traumatic origin of these three cases.

Two of my cases were women below middle age, but the remaining four were girls under eighteen years of age. In two of the six cases there was evidence of static incompetence of the feet. I have no reason to believe that this stood in any particular relationship to the condition which is here described.

Having observed six cases of this character in my own practice there would appear little doubt that the condition which I have described is not extremely infrequent. It is very likely that the similarity of symptoms to those of weak feet has caused it to be overlooked. While those cases in which there are no loose bodies will be relieved by the use of the felt pad if sufficiently long continued, the contrary will be true of the other cases. The cases with loose bodies will require arthrotomy as a rule. As in my first case, this may be unnecessary where the bodies are very few in number and very small.

It seems worthy of note that in my six cases only one foot has been the seat of this injury. While it is common enough to see only one foot affected in cases of metatarsal pain from static weakness, the contrary is the rule. This would seem, therefore, to be a point of some diagnostic importance.

Not a little interest attaches to the mechanism by which this injury to the foot takes place. Under normal circumstances the second metatarsal bone is slightly longer than the first. In the presence of a diminished power of toe flexion and especially of the great toe, it is apparent that forcible impact of the ball of the foot against the ground not sufficiently guarded by the flexor power of the toes will cause the distal end of the second metatarsal to bear the brunt of the blow. It seems likely to me that we have here the explanation of the mechanism of this injury.

7 MISCELLANEOUS DISORDERS

Gout: Hippocrates

Eunuchs do not take the gout nor become bald.
A woman does not take the gout, unless her menses are stopped.
A young man does not take the gout until he indulges in coition.

Gout: Thomas Sydenham, 1624-1689

Sydenham has a quality in common with Hippocrates: his writings cover a wide field with the accent on personal observation rather than quasi-scientific theorising, and, like Hippocrates, little is known of his life.

He was born at Winford Eagle, and studied at Oxford, but his studies were interrupted by the Civil Wars, during which he served in the Parliamentarian Army with the rank of Captain. On his return to Oxford he was created a Bachelor of Medicine by the Parliamentarian Chancellor of the University himself, by some very irregular procedure; he had only studied medicine for a few months altogether. He continued his studies at Montpellier, and then set up in practice in London.

He was a friend of Robert Boyle, the chemist, and John Locke. He wrote on the exanthems of childhood, and the use of quinine in malaria. He suffered from gout for many years, and his description of the disease is amongst his best work.

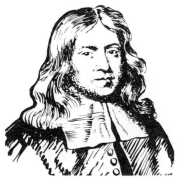

Gout: Thomas Sydenham, 1683

Either men will think that the nature of gout is wholly mysterious and incomprehensible, or that a man like myself who has suffered from it for thirty-four years, must be of a slow and sluggish disposition not to have discovered something respecting the nature and treatment of a disease so peculiarly his own. Be this as it may, I will give a bona fide account of what I know. The difficulties and refinements relating to the disease itself, and the method of its cure, I will leave for Time, the guide to truth, to clear up and explain.

Concerning this disease, in its most regular and typical state, I will first discourse; afterwards I will note its more irregular and uncertain phenomena. These occur when the unseasonable use of preposterous medicines has thrown it down from its original *status*. Also when the weakness and langour of the patient prevent it from rising to its proper and genuine symptoms. As often as gout is regular, it comes on thus. Towards the end of January or the beginning of February, suddenly and without any premonitory feelings, the disease breaks out. Its only forerunner is indigestion and crudity of the stomach, of which the patient labours some weeks before. His body feels swollen, heavy and windy—symptoms which increase until the fit breaks out. This is preceded a few days by torpor and a feeling of flatus along the legs and thighs. Besides this, there is a spasmodic affection, whilst the day before the fit the appetite is unnaturally hearty. The victim goes to bed and sleeps in good health. About two o'clock in the morning he is awakened by a severe pain in the great toe; more rarely in the heel, ankle or instep. This pain is like that of a dislocation, and yet the parts feel as if cold water were poured over them. Then follow chills and shivers and a little fever. The pain, which was at first moderate, becomes more intense. With its intensity the chills and shivers increase. After a time this comes to its height, accommodating itself to the bones and ligaments of the tarsus and metatarsus. Now it is a violent stretching and tearing of the ligaments—now it is a gnawing pain and now a pressure and tightening. So exquisite and lively meanwhile is the feeling of the part affected, that it cannot bear the weight of the bedclothes nor the jar of a person walking in the room. The night is passed in torture, sleeplessness, turning of the part affected, and perpetual change of posture; the tossing about of the body being as incessant as the pain of the tortured joint, and being worse as the fit comes on. Hence the vain effort, by change of posture, both in the body and limb affected, to obtain an abatement of the pain. This comes only towards the morning of the next day, such time being necessary for the moderate digestion of the peccant matter. The patient has a sudden and slight respite, which he falsely attributes to the last change of position. A gentle perspiration is succeeded by sleep. He wakes freer from pain, and finds the part recently swollen. Up to this time, the only visible swelling had been that of the veins of the affected joint. Next day (perhaps for the next two or three days), if the generation of the gouty matter had been abundant, the part affected is painful, getting worse towards evening and better towards morning. A few days after, the other foot swells, and suffers the same pains. The pain in the second foot attacked regulates the pain in the first one attacked. The more it is violent in the one, the more perfect is the abatement of suffering, and the return of strength in the other. Nevertheless, it brings on the same affliction here as it had brought on in the other foot, and that the same in duration and intensity. Sometimes, during the first days of the disease, the peccant matter is so exuberant, that one foot is insufficient for its discharge. It then attacks both, and that with equal violence. Generally, however, it takes the feet in succession. After it has attacked each foot, the fits become irregular, both as to the time of their accession and duration. One thing, however, is constant—the pain increases at night and remits in the morning. Now a series of lesser fits like these constitute a true attack of gout —long or short, according to the age of the patient. To suppose that an attack two or three months in length is all one fit is erroneous. It is rather a series of minor fits. Of these the latter is milder than the former, so that the peccant matter is discharged by degrees, and recovery follows. In strong constitutions, where the previous attacks have been few, a fortnight is the length of the attack. With age and impaired habits gout may last two months. With *very* advanced age, and in constitutions *very* much broken down by previous gout, the disease will hang on till the summer is far advanced. For the first fourteen days the urine is high-coloured, has a red sediment, and is loaded with gravel. Its amount is less than a third of what the patient drinks. During the same period the bowels are confined. Want of appetite, general chills towards evening, heaviness, and a troublesome feeling at the parts affected, attend the fit throughout. As the fit goes off, the foot itches intolerably, most between the toes; the cuticle scales off, and the feet desquamate, as if venomed. The disease being disposed of, the vigour and appetite of the patient return, and this in proportion to the violence of the last fits. In the same proportion the next fit either comes on or keeps off. Where one attack has been sharp, the next will take place that time next year—not earlier.

Gout produces calculus in the kidney. The patient has frequently to entertain the painful speculation as to whether gout or stone be the worst disease.

It makes life worse than death, and finally brings in death as a relief.

Dupuytren's Contracture

It is strange that a disease which occurs nowadays in about one in five of the population over the age of 60, and is so obvious to all, did not attract attention until the last century. Neither surgeon, artist, nor writer seem to have noticed the condition.

Dupuytren certainly gave the best account of it in a lecture at Hôtel Dieu, Paris, in 1833. This was published in the *Lancet* the following year, in accordance with Thomas Wakeley's plan to give publicity to the teachings of the men at the forefront of the profession. Apart from giving the condition the name of Dupuytren and acquainting doctors with the contracture, it encouraged one man, John Windsor, to look through lecture notes he had made as a student 25 years before. He had heard Henry Cline lecture on this in 1808.

"One or more of these tendinous columns of the aponeurosis palmaris sometimes becomes contracted and thickened; most generally only one is affected, but sometimes more and proportionably so many fingers are bent into the palm of the hand. The treatment is easy and efficacious; it consists in cutting through the aponeurosis with a common knife. In performing the operation, in order to avoid the blood vessels and nerves underneath, the fingers or finger may be kept extended afterwards by a splint, for the flexor muscle has in some degree become shortened and without this the disease might be reproduced."

Astley Cooper, too, recognised the condition, writing about it in his Treatise on dislocations and fractures of the joints in 1822:-

"The fingers are sometimes contracted in a similar manner, by a chronic inflammation of the thecae, and the aponeurosis of the palm of the hand, from excessive action of the hand in the use of the hammer, the oar, ploughing, etc., etc. When the thecae is contracted, nothing should be attempted for the patient's relief, as no operation or other means will succeed; but when the aponeurosis is the cause of the contraction and the contracted band is narrow, it may be with advantage divided by a pointed bistory, introduced through a very small wound in the integument. The finger is then extended and a splint is applied to preserve it in the straight position."

Dupuytren: 1833

*Permanent Retraction of the Fingers, Produced by
an Affection of the Palmar Fascia*

Retraction of the fingers, Gentlemen, and particularly that of the ring-finger, has been observed for many years, but it is only very lately that the cause of this deformity has been investigated with success.

The greater number of individuals affected by this disease have been obliged to make efforts with the palm of the hand, or frequently to handle hard bodies. Thus the wine-merchant and coachman of whom we shall presently speak were obliged, the one to perforate continually the casks with a gimlet, the other to ply his whip unceasingly on the backs of his jaded horses; it is also seen in masons who lift stones with the extremities of the fingers, in ploughmen, &c.; hence we see that the disease occurs most frequently in those who are forced in working to make the palm of the hand a *point d'appui*. Individuals who are predisposed to the disease of which we speak, perceive that they extend the fingers of the injured hand with less facility than usual; the ring-finger soon begins to contract; the deformity first attacks the proximal phalanx, and the others follow its movement: as the disease advances, the finger becomes more contracted, and the flexion of the two neighbouring fingers begins to be remarked. We do not feel any nodosity in front of the chord which runs along the palmar surface of the ring-finger; the two last phalanges are straight and movable at this period; and the proximal one is bent nearly at a right angle on the metacarpal bone, but still retains some motion; in this state it cannot be brought to its original position by the most violent effort. A person attacked by this infirmity attached to his finger a weight amounting to 150 pounds, without influencing in the least the degree of flexion. When the ring-finger is flexed to a great degree, the skin presents various folds, the convexity of which looks towards the articulation of the wrist.

But you may ask, what are the inconveniences of this affection? As the ring-finger cannot be extended, the motion of the two neighbouring fingers is much limited; the patient can only seize a very small body; if he attempt to grasp it strongly, he feels great pain; the very act of catching any body is painful. A man, who had been for a long time affected with this disease, happened to die. I had kept my eye on him for some years, and was determined not to lose this opportunity of investigation. Accordingly I possessed myself of the arm of this man, had the state of parts accurately drawn by an artist, and then proceeded to dissect them. When the skin was removed from the palmar surface of the hand and fingers, the folds which I have before noticed, disappeared altogether. It was evident then that the folded arrangement of the skin during life depended on some other affection; but what was this? The dissection was continued by exposing the palmar fascia, and I was astonished to perceive that this fascia was tense, retracted, and shortened. From its lower portion were given off kinds of chords, which passed to the diseased finger. In flexing and extending the fingers, I could clearly see that the fascia underwent a sort of tension, or crackling; this was a trace of light, and made me suspect that the aponeurosis had some connexion with the complaint. But the precise point affected remained to be discovered. I cut through the prolongations extending from the fascia to the fingers; the state of contraction immediately ceased, and the slightest effort was sufficient to bring them to complete extension; the tendons were all sound, and the sheaths had not been opened; but in order to leave no doubt on the subject, I examined the tendons with care. Their surfaces were smooth, and they enjoyed their usual degree of motion; the joints also were in a healthy state, the bones were neither swollen nor changed in any degree. I could distinguish no alteration of the articular surfaces or ligaments. The synovial membranes, the synovial cartilages, all were sound. It was, therefore, natural to conclude that the disease commenced in an exaggerated tension of the palmar fascia, which depended on the violent or long-continued action of some hard body on the palm of the hand.

CASES OF CONTRACTION OF THE RING AND LITTLE FINGERS COM-
PLETELY CURED BY DIVISION OF THE PALMAR APONEUROSIS

Case 1.—In 1811, M. L., wine-merchant, having received from the South a great deal of wine, was desirous to assist his workmen in arranging the casks in the store. While endeavouring to raise one of the casks, which was very heavy, by placing his hand under the edge of the stave, he felt a sensation of cracking and a slight pain in the palm of his hand. For some time the part remained stiff and sensible, but these symptoms soon went off, and he paid little attention to the state of his hand. The accident was nearly forgotten, when he perceived that the ring-finger commenced to contract towards the palm of his hand, and could not be extended as much as the other fingers. As there was no pain, he neglected this slight deformity. By degrees the disease advanced, and made a sensible progress each year, so that in 1831 the little and ring fingers were completely flexed, and applied to the palm of the hand; the second phalanx was folded on the first and the extremity of the third applied to the middle of the ulnar edge of the palmar surface. The small finger was firmly flexed on the palm of the hand; and the skin of this part was folded, and dragged towards the retracted fingers.

The patient, annoyed by seeing this deformity getting daily worse, consulted several surgeons, who all said that the disease existed in the flexor tendons, and advised their section as the only remedy; but some would cut both tendons, whilst others proposed to divide only one.

The moment I saw the man's hand I recognized the affection of the palmar fascia, declared the disease was not situated in the tendons, and that a few incisions practised in the aponeurosis would be sufficient to restore entire freedom of motion to the finger.

Operation: The hand of the patient being firmly fixed, I commenced the operation by making a transverse incision nearly an inch long, opposite the metacarpophalangeal articulation of the ring finger; the bistoury divided first the skin and then the palmar fascia, with a crackling sound perceptible to the ear; after this incision the ring-finger recovered its position and could be extended nearly as completely as ever. As I was desirous to spare the patient the pain of a new incision, I attempted to prolong the division of the fascia by gliding the bistoury deeply under the skin towards the ulnar edge of the hand, in order to free, if possible, the little finger, but this attempt failed. I was in consequence obliged to make another transverse incision opposite the articulation of the first and second phalanx of the little finger, which enabled me to detach it from the palm of the hand, but the rest of the finger remained obstinately fixed towards this part. A new incision, however, divided the skin and fascia opposite the metacarpal joint of the finger, to give it some slight liberty; finally, a third transverse cut was made opposite the middle of the first phalanx, and immediately extension of the finger was easily accomplished; this proved clearly that the last incision had divided the point of insertion of the fascial process. The wounds were simply dressed with dry lint, and the fingers kept in a state of extension by a suitable apparatus.

Progress of the case.—Next day, little pain; merely some uneasiness from the continued extension. On the following day the back of the hand was slightly oedematous from the pressure of the apparatus, which was clumsily made; another was applied, but the state of irritation continued, great pain set in, and the hand became much swollen. Not wishing to remove the machine applied to extend the fingers, I ordered the hand to be bathed continually with Goulard's solution, which gave considerable relief. On the 15th the lint was removed, and we found some suppuration had set in; the hand was still swollen and painful. Extension was continued to the same degree as formerly, and the cold lotion applied. On the 16th the swelling had abated considerably, the fingers remained stiff, and suppuration was fully established. 17th. The symptoms were more favourable, and the extension could be increased somewhat without determining any pain. Finally, in the course of some days the swelling of the hand disappeared, and the wounds were healed on the 2nd of July.

The cause of this slowness in the cicatrization depended, without doubt, on the forced extension in which the fingers were constantly kept. The patient continued to carry the apparatus for another month, in order to oppose the reunion of the edges of the divided fascia; and when at length this was removed, we had the satisfaction of seeing that he could flex his fingers with facility, and that the stiffness which remained was only due to the forced extension in which the articulations were held for so long a time; but this rigidity disappeared when the patient had, for a short time resumed his accustomed exercises.

Remarks.—This case can leave no doubt of the nature of the disease; but we may be inclined to ask, how can the palmar fascia determine similar effects? To answer this question, we must recall to your memory a few anatomical particulars concerning this fibrous envelope. The superficial palmar fascia is partly formed by the expansion of the tendon of the palmaris *longus*, and of the anterior portion of the annular ligament of the wrist. Though very strong in its origin, it thins by degrees, and sends off from its inferior margin four fibrous slips, which pass towards the inferior extremity of the four last metacarpal bones; here each of these slips bifurcates for the passage of the flexor tendons, and each branch of the bifurcated slip passes on to be attached to the *side*, and not to the front, of the phalanx, as most anatomists have thought. These are the slips of fascia which should be cut, whenever the operation becomes necessary. When we dissect off the skin from the fascia beneath, we find a certain difficulty in separating it, because the cellular tissue is dense, and because various fibrous filaments pass from the fascia into the integument; these adhesions explain readily the wrinkled state of the skin, and its motion. At first sight we might be inclined to dread cutting the nerves and vessels of the finger, but these parts are well protected by a kind of bridge formed by the contracted fibres, and run no risk of being divided.

The uses commonly attributed to the palmar fascia are to sustain the tendons of the flexor muscles, to strengthen the arch of the hand, and protect the different vessels and nerves there contained; but in addition to these, it tends constantly to bring the fingers to a state of demiflexion; which is their state of repose, and it is nothing more than the excess of this function, produced by disease, which gives rise to the deformity of which I now speak.

Case 2.—The subject of this operation was a coachman aged about 40. Several years back his fingers began to contract, especially the ring-finger. When he came to the Hôtel Dieu, the fingers were so much flexed that they nearly touched the palm of the hand; and this part formed numerous folds of skin, the convexity of which was turned towards the fingers. When we attempted to extend the fingers, we felt a chord stretching from them to the palm of the hand; both hands were affected by the disease, which could not be mistaken, from its history, and the symptoms before us. When the hand was seized, and the fingers moved, the tension of the fascia became manifest; I immediately divided with a curved bistoury the skin and fascia by two incisions, one at the base of the ring-finger, in order to cut the two slips of fascia passing to it; the second at about an inch and a quarter below the other, in the palm of the hand, in order to divide this prolongation, a second time, and at the point where its base joined the palmar aponeurosis. After three incisions the ring-finger recovered very nearly its normal position; though little blood was lost the patient himself felt weak, I therefore deferred operating on the left hand until another day. It is unnecessary to pursue the history of this case any further, as the treatment and success were exactly similar to the case already mentioned to you.

Concluding Remarks.—The facts which you have just heard, Gentlemen, establish, incontrovertibly, that retraction of the fingers depends, in these cases, on a retraction of the palmar fascia, and, finally, that this disease may be cured by the transverse sections of these slips, and of the fascia which furnishes them. These facts, are not, indeed, sufficient to establish any general doctrine, but they will not fail to awaken the attention of practitioners; and it is, I hope, probable that these hints may become useful to science and humanity, in multiplying observations on the cause, symptoms, and treatment of this disease. But we should remark, that all analogous cases do not strictly resemble one another, that various methods of cure shall be applied to various diseases, and that the very best may lose their reputation by being applied without care or discrimination; such, for example, would be the fate of the method I have indicated, if it were employed by retraction of the fingers caused by gout, rheumatism, whitlow, or other similar diseases.

de Quervain's Stenosing Tenovaginitis: Fritz de Quervain, 1868-1940

De Quervain was a most distinguished general surgeon and succeeded Kocher as Professor of Surgery at Berne. He was born at Sion in the Valais Canton of Switzerland, where his father was pastor. After studying at Berne, he settled as a surgeon in the watch-making district of La Chaux-de-Fonds. After eight years he returned to the University as Reader in Surgery under Kocher, becoming involved in the enormous programme of clinical and scientific work on goitre. He was responsible for the introduction of iodised table salt. His interests were very wide and he made contributions to most branches of surgery.

Grey Turner visited his clinic in 1908 and was vividly struck by his resource and imagination.

"It was a badly united fracture of the femur and he was finding difficulty in getting correct alignment and in fixing the fragments. In the middle of the operation, and apparently without premeditation, he sent for an old-fashioned vulcanite pessary. This he heated and moulded into a sort of angulated peg which fitted into the medullary cavities of the bone ends and served to give stability to the fragments while the wound was closed and the limb put up in a fixation apparatus."

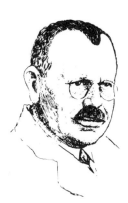

Concerning a Form of Chronic Tenovaginitis, by F. de Quervain, 1895

Although chronic inflammation of tendon sheaths is rightly and increasingly being regarded as due to tuberculosis, there are forms which cannot be classified as tuberculous either by their clinical appearance or by their anatomical situation. It may therefore seem right to report a series of cases, which, though having an affinity to tenosynovitis sicca, show significant differences from the accepted pattern and in which surgical intervention proved profitable.

Mrs. L., 55 years old. Besides keeping house she worked at gathering wood and in October 1893 she observed that movement of the right thumb was gradually becoming painful. The pain was chiefly localised to the distal end of the radius and radiated from there in to the fore-arm; on occasions it became so acute that the patient was unable to make gripping movements. This considerably interfered with her work. At first she did not observe any swelling, reddening of the skin, or crepitation. Only after several months did she think she could notice some slight swelling. Although she rubbed in spirit of camphor and applied warm compresses the complaint became worse rather than better; in February 1894 she decided to visit the surgical clinic. At that time her condition was as follows:-

She exhibited no general signs of tuberculosis, syphilis, or gout. Movement of the right thumb was painful as described above. Palpation of the tendon sheaths or tendons in question was normal apart from slight circumscribed thickening of the retinaculum overlying the extensor pollicis brevis and abductor pollicis longus at the lower end of the radius. This tendon sheath compartment was noticeably tender on palpation by contrast with the rest of the tendon sheath. There was no crepitation nor was there any motor disturbance in the sense of triggering. From her condition it could be assumed that this was not tuberculous and it was equally certain that it was not a form of gouty arthritis. It seemed most likely that it was a thickening of the tendon sheath at a specific point, i.e. at the fibrous extensor tunnel roofed by the extensor retinaculum. The functional disturbance was produced by an increase of friction at this point.

As she gave no report of any aetiologically significant trauma, the most likely cause was prolonged overstraining of the thumb, possibly connected with a "rheumatic" disposition, however indeterminate this may be.

On 7 March 1894, setting out with the idea that stenosis was the cause of the condition, I excised (under cocaine anaesthesia) the common tunnel of extensor pollicis brevis and abductor pollicis longus over a length of one centimeter, laying the tendons open to the subcutaneous tissue. The outer surface of the synovium showed not the slightest change; there was no effusion of fibrin, etc., and the underlying bone was sound. Only the excised tunnel of the tendon sheath seemed to show a certain thickening which was hard to define.

After the operation the pain which the patient had previously felt disappeared, and, after the incision had healed per primam, she began to use her thumb again without trouble. A report on 7th March 1895 shows that the patient remained perfectly well and the lack of the tendon sheath tunnel caused her no disturbance.

He operated on a further case and describes three others seen by a colleague. On the basis of these cases he draws a clinical picture of the disorder.

The patients feel more or less acute pain when moving the thumb; this radiates from the wrist to the thumb and the forearm and is of such degree that often they cannot continue to hold an object that they have picked up. Palpation shows either nothing or slight thickening of the tendon sheath tunnel at the distal end of the radius, which is in every case definitely tender to touch, whereas the rest of the tendon sheath is either less tender or not tender at all. This affection is always chronic.

De Quervain wondered why this should occur. Perhaps it is because the thumb is the most used digit and the radial styloid area is liable to injury. Kocher wrote to him about the condition and took the view that it began as an occupational hypertrophy of the tunnel. He compared it with Neal-aton's description of trigger finger but observed that, for no very obvious reason, the secondary nodule in the tendon was absent. De Quervain, too, thought that the thickening of the tendon sheath or of its synovial lining was responsible for the condition and that the friction generated by the stenosis aggravated it.

Apart from the rest he thought that surgery was the most rewarding method of treatment. He suggested a 4 centimetre incision in the line of the tendons, taking care to avoid the radial nerve. The roof of the tunnel should then be removed.

Vertebra Plana: Jacques Calvé, 1875-1954

Calvé studied in Paris as an orthopaedic surgeon and then worked in Berck with Dr. V. Menard. The Hospital was situated on the north coastline of France and had 1,100 beds for bone and joint tuberculosis to cater for some of the needs of Paris. When Calvé joined the hospital an X-ray machine was purchased, and he found that 10 children out of 500 with hip disease were in fact suffering from coxa plana.

He raised money from the Americans, and built a new hospital and trade school for children from the war-torn Channel region. He married an American. His main interest was tuberculosis, but, as so often happens, this is not his claim to fame. He described two of the 'flat' diseases—coxa plana in 1910, and vertebra plana in 1925.

He was a gracious, kindly man, and was a friend of Robert Jones.

1925

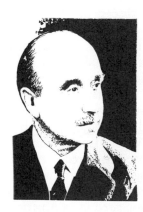

A LOCALISED AFFECTION OF THE SPINE SUGGESTING OSTEOCHONDRITIS OF THE VERTEBRAL BODY, WITH THE CLINICAL ASPECT OF POTT'S DISEASE

by Jacques Calvé, M.D., Berck, France

Chirurgien en Chef de la Fondation Franco-Américaine de Berck Plage, France

In this paper are submitted two observations, one of a case of my own, and one a case of my friend, Dr. Brackett, of Boston, who has been good enough to allow me to use the notes and illustrations of his case. They both occurred in patients in private practice and were observed carefully from the time of their first symptoms until their evident cure. Both cases were believed, during their entire evolution, to be Pott's disease, and were treated as such.

Observation 1.—P F., 2½ years of age. Onset: November, 1921, insidious, gradual, accompanied by pain in the back, and stiffness, with the appearance of a small knuckle in the dorsal region which rapidly increased. Parents consulted a specialist, who made the diagnosis of Pott's disease and sent the child to the Riviera. The case came under my observation for the first time in May, 1922, six months after the onset. At this time there were the usual symptoms of Pott's disease with a sharp knuckle. The child was difficult to manage and, the diagnosis appearing evident, it did not seem necessary to have an X-ray picture taken at that time, and the case was treated at Berck by hyperextension in a recumbent position until January, 1924. The knuckle disappeared progressively, no abscess threatened at any time, nor were there any symptoms, at any time, suggesting compression of the spinal cord. The child made a recovery without deformity and now walks like a normal child, and is wearing, at present, a celluloid jacket as a matter of protection.

Observation 2.—F. M., 7 years of age. Patient presented usual symptoms of an early spinal tuberculosis. No history of fall or injury other than those incident to the life of a healthy and active boy. There were early premonitory symptoms of tiredness, disinclination for prolonged play, etc., but not sufficient to call attention to them at the time; later, very marked sensitiveness to all motion, night cries, spasm with rigid spine, forward stoop in standing, and a small sharp knuckle of one spinous process. Treatment by plaster jacket at first, and with recumbency for several months, then gradual resumption of limited activity. After two or three months pain and sensitiveness entirely disappeared, and the patient has had no symptoms since. For the past three years he has lived the active life of a normal boy, taking part in games, but still wearing the plaster jacket. Between the first and second year the knuckle disappeared; none can be seen now, but one spinal process can be felt to be slightly prominent.

As seen from a clinical point of view, these were cases of dorsal Pott's disease. Neither developed an abscess or symptoms of spinal cord compression, the evolution was rapid, and the disease was, perhaps, cured in a shorter period than usual. Nevertheless, at the time this did not seem a sufficient reason for doubting the diagnosis of the tubercular nature of the affection, nor was there any doubt of the diagnosis until the evidence of the first roentgenograms was considered. As has already been stated, my patient was extremely difficult to manage, which prevented a roentgenogram being taken at the beginning of the treatment. When, from a clinical point of view, it was considered that the disease was cured, a roentgenogram was taken to confirm this clinical diagnosis of cure, and at once the abnormal aspect of the picture was apparent and raised a doubt of the original diagnosis. As there had appeared in an American journal at the same period a roentgenogram of the case treated by Dr. Brackett, which bore a striking resemblance to that of my own case, I obtained a picture of this case.

A study of the two roentgenograms shows, in my opinion, the

difference between them and pictures taken of a case of true Pott's disease.

1. In these two cases the lesion attacks only one vertebra (there is but one pedicle). The lamellar aspect of the osseus nucleus, regular in one case, irregular in the other, and slightly wedge-shaped, can be found in Pott's disease (especially in the lumbar region), but in Pott's disease there are always at least two pedicles, at least two of the vertebrae being affected or destroyed. This cuneiform shape always indicates the total destruction of the inter-vertebral disc.

2. In striking contrast here is the absolutely intact condition of the adjacent discs above and below the diseased vertebra.

3. The cartilage is thicker and there is a neoformation of this tissue. The transparent part above and below the lamellar osseous nucleus is at least a third higher than it is normally. (This is never seen in tuberculosis, which is markedly destructive of cartilage tissue).

4. Greater opacity is to be remarked, which indicates that the bone density has increased. This characteristic is especially noted in the observation of Case 2, but is also perceptible in Case 1.

With the evidence of this abnormal characteristic, tubercular tests were made under such conditions that all possibility of a mistake was eliminated in both cases. The tests were negative. The Wassermann test was also made and resulted in negative findings in both cases. We are, therfore, justified in ruling out a diagnosis of tubercular infection in either of these two cases, and this observation, combined with the similarity of the roentgenograms, justifies the consideration of these two cases in the same category. It might seem presumptuous on my part to suggest a pathologic entity from the observation of two cases only, but one may advance a suppositional diagnosis while waiting for other observations to corroborate these findings, and it is hoped that other observations will be stimulated by this short paper.

In what type of disease can these two cases be catalogued? Tuberculosis and syphilis must be eliminated. Neither can trau-matism (that is Kümmel's disease) be suspected, for in both cases the parents were positive that there had been no serious injury or fall previous to the first symptoms. The idea of congenital mal-formation must also be eliminated.

The clinical history of both cases is manifestly and incontestably that of an affection developed after birth. The cases also show a regeneration of bone in the later stages of the convalescence, and in Case 2, an increase could be observed in roentgenograms taken two or three years apart. An infectious origin is, on the other hand, more probable. In Case 2 there were no observations on this point. In Case 1 the patient had an attack of enteritis with fever at the time the back symptoms appeared. It is impossible not to recognise by the roentgenograms and the clinical manifestations some connection between these two cases and coxa plana, Legg-Calvé's disease, infantile osteochondritis of the hip, as well as Koehler's disease. Here is also found the reverse of the usual formula (upon which I have already insisted in reference to coxa plana) which may be thus expressed: "less bone, more cartilage." In this the same density of bony substance is found which is the rule in Koehler's disease.

The affection which I have just submitted to you is, I believe, to the spinal column what coxa plana is to the hip, and what Koehler's disease is to the foot.

Ganglion: Paul of Aegina, 625-690

Paul was born on the island of Aegina and practised in Alexandria.

His book, *The Epitome of Medicine*, occupied seven volumes, and, though not original, it remained standard reading for a long while, as it covered everything that was known about medicine and surgery at that time. His section on fractures is little different to Hippocrates.

Paul was the last of the Byzantine doctors and continued to work in Alexandria after the Arab invasion. After him Arabic medicine dominated Western civilisation for nearly 400 years during the Dark Ages.

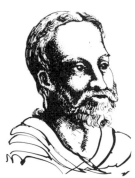

Paul of Aegina: 7th Century

ON GANGLION

A ganglion is a round tumour of a tendon, arising from a blow or violent exercise, being formed most frequently about the wrist, ankles, and the parts about a joint which are much moved, but likewise in the other parts. It is attended with a swelling, which is free from discoloration, unyielding, and without pain, but if strongly pressed upon it has a dull feeling. It is not deep-seated, but takes its origin under the skin, and may be moved laterally, but cannot by any means be forced forwards and backwards. Those then which form in the legs, arms, and extremities it is not safe to cut out, for there is danger lest the part be mutilated. But those about the head or forehead we operate upon by dividing the skin with a scalpel, and if the tumours be small, seizing them with a flesh forceps and cutting them out by the roots. But if they are larger, we transfix them with hooks, and remove them by dissecting them from the skin, and uniting the lips with sutures, and complete the cure by the treatment applicable to fresh wounds.

Ankylosing Spondylitis

At the end of the seventeenth century, Bernard Connor, an Irishman who became physician to the King of Poland and died of malaria at the age of 32 in London, came across "an extraordinary human skeleton, whose vertebrae of the back, the ribs, and several bones down to the os sacrum, were all firmly united into one solid bone, without jointing or cartilage."

He concluded that this person must have been incapable of motion, unable to bend or stretch, and that his respiration was limited. The dramatic picture of fully developed ankylosing spondylitis was the subject of several case histories. Delpeche in 1828 gives a good account, and Paget noticed it in 1877 (see page 22), but it was not until the late nineteenth century that much interest was aroused.

A. Strümpell, in 1884, wrote:-

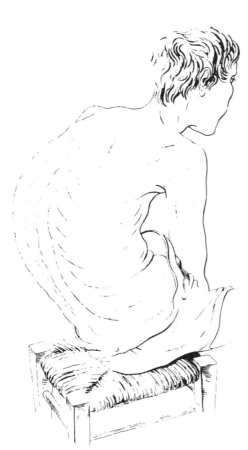

Ankylosing Spondylitis: Delpeche

"As a remarkable, and, it would seem, definite disease, we might now draw attention to a form of illness in which there supervenes, progressively and without pain, a complete ankylosis of the entire spine and both hip joints, in such a manner that the head, the trunk and the thighs become fused and completely rigid, while the other joints retain their normal mobility. It goes without saying that, as a result of this fusion, very definite alterations of posture and gait make their appearance. We ourselves have seen two identical cases of this singular condition."

Pierre Marie in 1898 gives a textbook description of the disorder. Eight years later he filled in the details in a paper with Léri. C. W. Buckley was first to call the disease ankylosing spondylitis in 1935.

Pierre Marie, 1853-1940

Pierre Marie was a great teacher. His square-cut hair, square-cut beard and striking personality gave him a severe, dignified and authoritarian manner in public, but at home, where he collected painting and sculpture, this thawed. He had no longing for honours or titles, being happy enough to devote his life to neurology and arouse the same enthusiasm in others.

Marie was born in Paris near Place de la Concorde when this had fields nearby. At his father's insistence he read law and was called to the bar, but then followed his own desire to study medicine. He became an intern under Charcot and continued to work for him for many years. In his doctoral thesis he first described the tremor of thyrotoxicosis. He had a succession of distinguished appointments—Physician at the Bicêtre, Professor of Pathological Anatomy, and Professor of Clinical Neurology at the Salpêtrière following Charcot and Déjerine.

Many of his original ideas were presented at his lectures and in consequence they were well attended. He kept up the Charcot tradition of attracting large numbers of post-graduate students.

His middle age was his most productive period and his old age was a succession of personal tragedies. His wife died, his daughter died of appendicitis and finally his son, who was studying botulism at the Institut Pasteur, contracted the disease and died.

What were Marie's contributions? Within three years of qualification he had described peroneal muscular atrophy. (Tooth, in this country, described it in the same year.) He made the first observation of acromegaly in 1886 and observed the pituitary tumour without realising its significance. Other workers showed that it was due to an eosinophil adenoma in 1909, but it was not until Evans and Long isolated the growth hormone in 1921 that the story was complete.

Marie described hypertrophic pulmonary osteo-arthropathy in 1890. In 1898 he published the first account of cranio-cleidal dysostosis and wrote the following account of ankylosing spondylitis. His only other contribution of interest to orthopaedic surgeons was his continued belief that poliomyelitis was infectious.

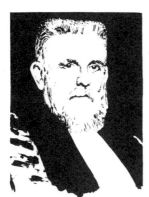

Pierre Marie on Spondylosis Rhizomélique: 1898

A particular characteristic of this disease is the occurrence of complete fusion of the spine together with a more or less pronounced ankylosis of the joints at the bases of the limbs, while the small joints remain unaffected.

We are going to examine each of the phrases of this definition separately:-

The Fusion of the Spine is complete, at least in the lower half; slightly higher, and especially in the cervical region, the spinal column may retain a certain mobility for some time. The rigidity thus produced is such that the spine would fracture rather than allow the slightest movement in it.

The position in which this fusion of the spine occurs is worth noting. It is not a question of a curviliginous Kyphosis comparable to those that may be seen in several other diseases; in rhizomelic spondylosis the kyphosis is above all due to a definite and rather acute bend at the cervical section of the spine, and also a little of the upper dorsal spine, while the lumbar and lower and middle dorsal sections of the spine often continue almost in a straight line. What considerably exaggerates the kyphotic appearance of these patients is the ankylosis of the hip joint in flexion, so that the trunk seems to be thrown further forward than it is in fact.

The fusion of the spine with the sacrum is complete—it seems that at this level even a bony proliferation may be formed; in particular one may encounter osteophytic prominences at the level of the sacro-iliac joint. Furthermore, the hyperostoses do not appear to be limited to the lower posterior section of the spine, for one finds, by feeling within the mouth, that bony protruberances on the anterior surfaces of the vertebral bodies are palpable through the posterior pharyngeal wall. It is most likely that the difficulty, which some of these patients experience when swallowing, is due to the irregularity at this level.

Ankylosis of the Joints of the Limbs. The joint which is most affected, and the only one which is really the site of complete ankylosis, is the hip joint. In this joint there may be complete loss of movement, with the joint fixed in some flexion and adduction.

The Scapulo-Humeral Joint is much less frequently affected than the hip joint and does not suffer comparable ankylosis. Nevertheless movements were considerably reduced in two of our patients. Neither of them can lift their arms above the horizontal; when they are told to put a hand on their head—if they can manage it—it is due to the kyphosis which pushes their head forward and to the swinging movement of the scapula. When these two patients carried out passive movements gross crepitus could be observed at the site of the acromio-coracoid arch.

The Knee is another joint in which symptoms may require study. At first sight movements appear to be completely normal and patients do not mention their knees; nevertheless if they are asked to bend their knees as much as possible, it can be seen that movement is limited to a greater or lesser extent; in no case is it sufficient for the heel to touch the buttock.

The other joints appear undamaged; their mobility is absolutely normal and contrasts with the ankylosis of the hip joint and the awkwardness of shoulder movement.

As for the fingers and hands, one must point out the obvious presence (in two patients) of the 'nodosities de Bouchard'.

The appearance of the patient is profoundly altered by a singular and very marked flattening of the pelvis and thorax. It is difficult to say whether the flattening of the pelvis is due only to atrophy of the buttocks or whether the bones themselves participate; this latter hypothesis is not unlikely. The thorax is, like the pelvis, flattened in the antero-posterior diameter; here, too, muscular wasting of the back muscles may play a certain part, though the skeleton shares in the deformity. This is very clear when one looks at the patient from the side.

In addition to this deformity there is extraordinary respiratory immobility of the chest; the ribs (except occasionally for the lowest ones) do not move during respiration, which is almost entirely abdominal.

As for the muscular atrophy: we would point out that, though it is very clear, it does not seem to us to be as pronounced as it may be in certain cases of monarticular arthritis.

Obviously such gross disease of many of the principal joints will lead to functional disabilities. In order to stand, the patients are forced to resort to a trick—they keep their knees in some flexion. Indeed, without this expedient, the trunk, leaning noticeably forwards as a result of the fixed, flexed hips, would bowl the patient over and make him incapable of keeping his balance. The flexion of the knee joint remedies this and compensates for the hip flexion. The occurrence of flexion at the two principal joints of the lower limbs has the result that these patients, on standing, resemble a letter Z. When they have to remain in this position for some time they are forced to make use of a stick, or else to lean forward with the hands resting on the front of the thighs.

In bed they cannot lie as they would like, for if they lay flat on their back in bed the fixed flexed spine would tend to lift up the pelvis and lower limbs. The only position in which one patient can get to sleep is on his side; another has constructed above his bed an iron bracket to which a sling is attached—this passes under his occiput, holding his head and shoulders well above the level of the bed, on which his lower limbs are resting.

As for walking: this too has a peculiar appearance because the hip joints are not functional. Progress forwards depends on movements at the knee and ankle joints. The patients look like wooden dolls, in which the leg movements occur about one transverse axis through the two knees. Though it is possible for them to walk unaided, they prefer to use two sticks or crutches because it is both difficult and painful.

It would be foolish to lay down any rules concerning the aetiology and natural history of the disease as we have seen only a small number of cases. However some points may be made at this stage.

All the cases I have been able to review have been men—is this simply a coincidence?

It is a disease which begins in early adult life, though it can begin in adolescence. Koehler had a case beginning over the age of fifty.

As for the actual commencement of the disease: the initial symptom appears to be pain, which started in the knee in two patients. Later they were seized with such severe pain in the sacro-coccygeal region, which lasted for months, that these poor patients could not remain in the sitting position.

It must be added that pain is an ordinary accompaniment of rhizomelic spondylosis; indeed one may sometimes observe spontaneous painful lumps on certain joints during its evolution; at other times with these cases the pains are unremitting. It is easy enough to reproduce them for a few minutes or a few hours, by insisting on an examination of the ankylosed joints, by changing the patient's chair or bed, or by making him perform unaccustomed movements.

As for the spinal rigidity: in two patients this has clearly advanced progressively from the sacrum to the cervical region; the hip joints seem to have been affected at the same time as the fusion of the lower regions of the spine.

It should be noted that in spite of the presence of pains which would seem to indicate an acute process, the joints have never shown the other characteristics of an acute or subacute arthritis (swelling, redness, heat); the process does not resemble acute articular rheumatism, nor deforming chronic rheumatism in its acute form. The tendency to ankylosis with deformity is predominant and unavoidable; in one patient complete ankylosis returned a few months after resection of part of the femoral neck and mobilisation of the joint.

PART THREE

PATHOLOGY

PATHOLOGY

Although the pathological anatomy of disorders of bone lent itself to early description and illustration, much still remains to be learnt about the mechanism of these changes.

Two of the best early nineteenth-century accounts of pathological changes and their production come from Dupuytren.

Congenital Dislocation of the Hip: Dupuytren: 1826

Dupuytren gives an excellent account of congenital dislocation of the hip. He considered its aetiology, drawing attention to its familial tendency, described its pathology very accurately and gave several case histories.

After considering several possible causes, such as violence, intra-uterine disease, faulty development of the os ilii, he wrote:-

> Is it not more probable that this displacement is accidental, and analogous in its nature, if not in its special cause, to those dislocations which occur during life from falls, blows, &c? But what, it may be asked again in answer to this hypothesis, could have been the effort or violence to have produced such a displacement? I will take the liberty of throwing out a remark which may, in some measure, be considered as supporting this explanation; it is this. The position of the lower extremities of the foetus in utero is such, that the thighs are very much bent on the belly, from which it follows that the heads of the thigh-bones are continuously pressing against the lower and back part of the capsular ligament—a circumstance which, though without effect in well-formed individuals, might, I apprehend, have an injurious influence in such as are weak, or of lax, unresisting fibre. If this premise is conceded, there is not much difficulty in imagining that dislocation may result; and the supposition is further strengthened by the fact that the most powerful of the muscles surrounding the articulation have a constant tendency to draw upwards the heads of the thigh-bones, as soon as they escape from the acetabula.
>
> I must remark that original or congenital dislocation of the thigh-bones is not so rare as may be supposed. I have met with as many as twenty cases in the course of eighteen years. Almost all the individuals who are affected with this deformity are females: indeed, out of twenty-six cases which I have examined, not more than two or three at most were males.

Case 1. *Original dislocation of the ossa femoris. Retention of urine, terminating fatally; autopsy.*—A man, 74 years of age, suffering from retention of urine, was admitted into the Hôtel-Dieu in February 1828. Several attempts had been made by different surgeons to pass a catheter, and M. Breschet had succeeded once, but failed a second time. I may just remark, in passing, that this case afforded an illustration of the importance of carrying the catheter along the upper wall of the urethra, to avoid the false passages, constrictions, and obstacles which are almost always found to exist at the lower part of this passage. On the admission of this patient, it was anticipated that he would not long survive, and as there were several peculiarities which suggested the probability of there being congenital dislocation of the thigh-bones, I felt considerable interest in the examination of the body, which the patient's death shortly afterwards afforded me an opportunity of prosecuting.

Autopsy.—In the first place it was observed that the thighs could not be separated as in abduction, without making them describe a segment of a large circle: the trochanters were much nearer to the crests of the ilia, and higher than natural; the heads of the bones were very much elevated, the knees inverted and the thighs shortened; in fact, there was a total change in the relations, direction and length of the limb. This was the consequence of the cavity destined by nature to receive the head of the bone being almost effaced, and of the latter being deformed. The upper part of each thigh was enlarged, the trunk curved backwards, and the belly protruded; the pelvis had almost lost the oblique bearing which is natural to it; the thighs were shortened, and the buttocks soft and flabby, which was explained by the approximated attachments of the great gluteal muscles, and the consequently relaxed conditions of their intermediate bellies. The gluteus medius was, on the contrary, distended and raised up, the gluteus minimus entirely wasted, and the pyramidalis, instead of being oblique in its direction as is normally the case, was quite horizontal: the gemelli and quadratus were distended, and the adductors were abridged of their natural length.

On the left side, the original cavity did not measure more than an inch at its greatest diameter; it was very shallow, rugged, and filled with a fatty substance of a yellowish colour, and almost of the fluidity of oil; its form was nearly an oval. The external iliac fossa presented, in front of the sciatic notch, a broad, shallow depression, lined by a thick glistening periosteum, which had almost the appearance of articular cartilage; it was on this that the head of the femur rested. The last-mentioned process itself was diminished in volume, a little flattened, irregular, and without any vestige to mark the attachment of the round ligament; it was, nevertheless, invested by articular cartilage which was thinner than natural. The fibrous capsule of the joint, which was in form exactly like a purse, was attached to the upper and lower borders of the original acetabulum, and was in place of an osseous cavity on the side it covered; its length was sufficient to allow the ascent of the head of the femur to the depression I have just described: the space over which it extended amounted to about three inches. This capsule was very thick, and almost as dense as the cartilage.

On the right side, the original cavity was a little larger, but its interior presented the same appearance as the other. The external iliac fossa, instead of exhibiting, as on the opposite side, a simple depression, presented, in front of the great sciatic notch, and nearly on a level with the space between the two anterior iliac spines, a broad and deep depression, with an osseous margin which was strongly marked, rough, and irregular. The head of the femur, which was larger than that of the other side, had likewise more nearly preserved its natural shape; but it was, as the left, invested by an imperfect articular cartilage, and both surfaces of the articulation were covered by synovial membrane. The orbicular ligament was not so thick as that of the opposite side, although its extent was not strictly limited to that of the circumference of the abnormal cavity. On this (the right) side, the head of the femur was supported by the osseous margin, whereas, on the left, the fibrous capsule was the only structure which, by its great strength and resistance, was effectively opposed to the weight of the body.

In addition to the above peculiarities there was very unusual mobility at the lumbo-sacral articulation; so that when the lower extremities and pelvis were fixed, the vertebral column could be moved freely upon the latter. The lax state of the intervertebral fibro-cartilage was the only recognisable cause of this singular mobility.

On the Formation of Callus; and on the Means of Remedying its Faulty or Misshapen Deposit: Dupuytren

There is probably no subject in pathological anatomy which has more largely exercised the sagacity of practical men and the imagination of theorists, without their having recourse to the aid of actual observation or experiment, than the question respecting the formation of callus. In modern times, two opinions in particular have been paramount, viz., those of Duhamel and Bordenave. The former of these attributed the consolidation of fractures to swelling of the periosteum and medullary membrane, to their extension from one fragment of the bone to the other, and ultimately to their reunion and ossification. According to him, this reunion was effected by a simple external annular deposit, or this was double, one division embracing the periphery of the fragment, whilst the other forced its way, like a peg, into the interior of the medullary canal. Bordenave's theory differed from this: he admitted that the reunion and consolidation of fractures are accomplished by a process analogous to that by which the healing of wounds in soft parts is effected. He thought he perceived cellular and vascular spots amongst the fragments of broken bone; and these, he conceived, coalesced, and afterwards became solid by the accumulation of phosphate of lime in their interior. John Hunter, again, ascribed all to the organisation of the blood which is effused around and between the fragments of bone; whilst Camper maintained that reunion is due to the formation of a double layer of callus, the external portion of which is adjacent to the periosteum; and the internal (an expansion of the inner osseous laminae) he describes as encroaching on the medullary canal.

These doctrines, with certain modifications, were generally received when I undertook, in 1808, to verify the opinions of Bordenave, which had been revived by Bichat. But I was much surprised, in examining the bodies of persons who had died after fractures, to find nothing which could be considered as confirmatory of the received opinions; and my further researches induced me to establish a theory, which was in part founded on that of Duhamel, but which involved the discovery of two new laws.

A natural distinction presents itself to the mind between the phenomena attendant on the deposit of callus in simple and complicated fractures; in the latter, where the displacement or destruction of texture is considerable, it is not the periosteum alone, but the filamentous tissue, ligaments, tendons, and even the muscles themselves which concur in the formation of callus.

In the second place, it was easy to perceive that Duhamel had stopped considerably short of the whole truth in his observations; he correctly described all that takes place in the periosteum and medullary membrane, and which constitutes the first stage in the curative process, but omits to notice that which invariably succeeds, and has for its seat the interval between the fragments; immediate reunion of the fracture, and progressive destruction of the first or preparative process, are effected by this second stage.

Convinced by my experiments that Nature never accomplishes the immediate union of a fracture, save by the formation of two successive deposits of callus, I have been induced to name one *provisional* and the other *permanent*. The former of these, which is usually perfected in about thirty to forty days, and which comprises the ossification due to the vessels of the periosteum, the filamentous tissue, sometimes even of the muscles, and of the medullary tissue, has not always strength enough (especially in oblique fractures) when the splints and other supports are removed, to resist the power of the muscles, or such passive force as may be applied, even to a moderate extent, to the seat of injury; and the brittleness of this provisional callus is such that the bone more readily yields at the point where it is deposited than at any other part. The second (permanent) callus, formed by the reunion of the surfaces of the fracture, possesses a solidity superior even to that of the bone itself, so that the latter would sooner break at any other point than where the former is deposited. The production and organisation of the permanent callus is never completed under eight, ten, or twelve months, a period which is further marked by the disappearance of the provisional callus, and the renewed continuity of the medullary canal.

The following are the principal phenomena which may be observed during the time that elapses between the occurrence of the fracture and the complete and exact reunion of the broken bone; their succession is so constant and unvarying, that they may be referred to *five different periods*. The *first* extends over the eight or ten days which immediately succeed the accident, and presents the following characters: at the moment that the fracture occurs, the periosteum and medullary membrane, the filamentous tissue, and sometimes even the muscles, are torn; blood escapes from the ruptured vessels, and surrounds the fragments, is poured into the medullary canal, and distends the neighbouring filamentous tissue. After a time the vessels retract, and their mouths are closed, the blood ceases to escape, and a mild inflammation is set up in all these parts. The filamentous tissue, reddened by a multitude of small vessels, becomes distended, condensed, and thickened, losing its elasticity, and acquiring a remarkable consistence; irregular prolongations are sent from it into the interstices of the muscles, by which their organisation is altered, and they are made to participate altogether or in part in the changes which are going on; their texture is transformed into one closely allied to the condensed filamentous, and they are united and confounded with the periosteum, which, in turn, is also thickened by a network of delicate red vessels distributed over its surface. The medulla being broken through and mingled with blood, at first swells out and hardens, and subsequently becomes of a greyish white colour. The medullary canal is contracted in its diameter by the encroachment of the thickened lining membrane, which assumes a reddish, fleshy or pulpy appearance, resulting from a sort of gelatinous infiltration. The coagulum which results from the primary extravasation is absorbed and disappears. A stringy and viscid matter sometimes presenting a gelatinous appearance, is poured out between the ends of the bone; occasionally likewise a reddish substance is developed in the same position, springing from the inequalities which present themselves; they grow and extend towards each other in the form of rosy points, and ultimately meet and interlace with each other. This production, the nature of which is but little understood, never acquires any great amount of thickness or density; it becomes continuous internally with the medullary membrane, and externally is identified with the congested soft parts; it is not always met with, and then the viscid and gelatinous matter of which mention has been made is alone present. Both of these structures, whether found separately or together, appear to play an important part in the production of the callus, but of the permanent callus only. The fragments of the bone are, in short, surrounded by the gorged soft parts, which are converted into a homogeneous tissue of a lardaceous consistence and red colour, but varying in intensity.

The *second period* then commences, and comprises the interval between the tenth or twelfth day and the twentieth or twenty-fifth. The gorged condition of the surrounding soft parts diminishes, the muscular tissue resumes its distinctive characteristics, but the filamentous tissue continues condensed. The tumefaction is more concentrated immediately about the fracture, and gradually assumes a more circumscribed character, until it forms a distinct tumour isolated from all surrounding structures, not even excepting the tendons, which play in grooves channeled for them along its surface, or in perfect canals traversing its structure; such is the *callus*. This tumour is thicker on a level with the fracture than at any other point, and insensibly diminishes in density on either of the fragments. Its tissue is homogeneous, its colour white or whitish, its consistence firm, and its resistance analogous to that of the fibrocartilages, giving out a similar sound when cut with a sharp knife. The deepest part of this structure, that which is formed by and continuous with the periosteum, is found to contract more close adhesions to the bones the nearer it approaches to the fracture, at which point it is difficult to separate them. If, however, this separation is effected with the aid of the handle of a scalpel, it is perceived that they are formed of longitudinal fibres parallel to those of the bones, and analogous to the fibre of tendons; or they may exist in the form of cartilaginous or osseous striæ, according to the more or less advanced condition of the provisional callus. Towards the extremities of the tumour formed by the callus, the periosteum becomes more distinct and easy to detach from the bone. The medullary membrane, swollen, tumid, and identified with the matter by which it is infiltrated, sometimes obliterates the canal, not only on a level with the fracture, but for some distance on either side of it; thus filling up the space usually occupied by the medulla, which is proportionately diminished in quantity; the cylinder which it forms passes rapidly into a cartilaginous state, and still more quickly into bone, becoming identified with the seat of fracture with the whitish, rosy, red or violet-coloured, viscid, or gelatinous substance as the case may be, which is interposed between the fragments; on the other hand, it is lost in the callus externally. Whilst in this condition it is still possible for the callus to yield opposite the fracture, but crepitus is rarely reproduced.

The *third period* extends from the twentieth or twenty-fifth day to the thirtieth, fortieth, or sixtieth, according to the rapidity of the work of reproduction, and the age, constitution, and health of the patient. The conversion into cartilage commences at the centre of the tumour, and proceeds towards its circumference, and ossification speedily succeeds; thus little by little, the whole mass of callus becomes converted into bone. The periosteum, which is abnormally thick, then ceases to present any trace of the solution of continuity to which it had been subjected; and the muscles and tendons become free, though their natural mobility is not quite restored, on account of the induration of the filamentous tissue. If, at this epoch, a section of the callus is made, the fractured ends of the bone are still found moveable on each other, the condition of the intermediate substance not being as yet sensibly changed; and the tissue of the callus presents all the characteristics of the spongy texture of bone.

The *fourth period* includes the interval between the fiftieth or sixtieth day and the fifth or sixth month. The substance of the provisional callus becomes condensed, and passes from the condition of a spongy to that of a compact tissue, and the medullary canal is obliterated by osseous matter of greater or less density. The substance intervening between the fragments is reduced to a mere line of a different colour from the bone itself; it gradually assumes more consistence, loses its colour, and ultimately, towards the end of this period, becomes ossified: the definitive or, permanent callus is then formed.

The *fifth* and *last period* embraces all the time which elapses between the fourth or sixth, and the eighth, tenth, or twelfth, months. The temporary callus gradually diminishes in thickness, and at last disappears; the periosteum recovers its natural texture and density, and the muscles and tendons are restored to perfect liberty; the internal deposit of bone disappears, and the canal is insensibly re-established; the medullary membrane is repaired, and the medulla is reproduced. The process of consolidation is then completed.

The foregoing details are of great practical importance, as they indicate the precautions it is necessary to take during the progress of the cure of fractures generally, and more especially of oblique fractures affecting the long bones, of those of the cervix femoris, the patella, the olecranon, and the os calcis; in reference to which they offer a satisfactory explanation of the difficulty attending the cure, and of the giving way of the fractured ends resulting from the feeble resistance of the provisional callus. One of the most interesting and useful consequences of this doctrine is the correction of the deformed union of fractures, before the period of formation of the permanent callus.

PART FOUR

PHYSICAL SIGNS

Heberden's Nodes: William Heberden, 1710-1801

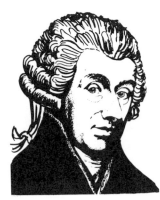

"Was born in London in the year 1710, and received the early part of his education in that city. At the close of the year 1724 he was sent to St. John's College in Cambridge and six years after was elected a Fellow. From that time he directed his attention to the study of medicine, which he pursued partly at Cambridge and partly in London. Having taken his degree of Doctor of Physic he practised in the University for about ten years, and during that time read every year a course of lectures on the Materia Medica. In the year 1746 he became a Fellow of the Royal College of Physicians, and two years afterwards, leaving Cambridge, he settled in London and was elected into the Royal Society. He very soon got into great business, which he followed with unremitting attention above thirty years, till it seemed prudent to withdraw a little from the fatigues of his profession. He therefore purchased a house at Windsor, to which he used ever afterwards to retire during some of the summer months; but returned to London in the winter, and still continued to visit the sick for many years.

In 1766 he recommended to the College of Physicians the first design of the Medical Transactions, in which he proposed to collect together such observations as might have occurred to any of their body, and were likely to illustrate the history or cure of diseases. The plan was soon adopted, and three volumes have successively been laid before the public. In 1778 the Royal Society of Medicine in Paris chose him into the number of their Associates. Besides the observations contained in the present volume, Doctor Heberden was the author of several papers in the Medical Transactions, and of some in the Philosophical Transactions af the Royal Society. He declined all professional business several years before his death, which was mercifully postponed till the year 1801, when he was advancing to the age of ninety-one.

From his early youth he had always entertained a deep sense of religion, a consummate love of virtue, an ardent thirst after knowledge, and an earnest desire to promote the welfare and happiness of mankind. By these qualities, accompanied with great sweetness of manners, he acquired the love and esteem of all good men, in a degree which perhaps very few have experienced; and after passing an active life with the uniform testimony of good conscience, he became an eminent example of its influence, in the cheerfulness and serenity of his latest age."

Biographical Notes by his Son.

Digitorum Nodi 1802

What are those little hard knobs, about the size of a small pea, which are frequently seen upon the fingers, particularly a little below the top, near the joint? They have no connection with the gout, being found in persons who never had it: they continue for life; and being hardly ever attended with pain, or disposed to become sores, are rather unsightly than inconvenient, though they must be some little hindrance to the free use of the fingers.

Thomas' Hip Flexion Test: 1876

Hugh Owen Thomas was very aware that chronic joint disease produced deformity, though he had neither the inclination, nor the means at that time, to discover the aetiology in any particular case. Not only was deformity a diagnostic aid, but it was the most important element to correct by treatment. Most of the cases of hip disease that he encountered were of tuberculous origin; he used this test to recognise them and assess their progress.

The diagnostic method which I shall demonstrate is of value to the surgeon in the case of children in particular, as he can get all the information in defiance of the struggles of the patient, and without administering an anaesthetic, and it enables him to estimate how long a time the patient has been suffering, whether one week or twelve months. For all practical purposes the symptoms are often as well defined in twelve months as they are in as many years.

Having undressed the patient and laid him on his back upon a table or other hard plane surface, the surgeon takes the sound limb and flexes it, so that the knee joint is in contact with the chest. Thus he makes certain that the spine and back of the pelvis are lying flat on the table; an assistant maintains the sound limb in this flexed position; the patient is then urged to extend, as far as he is able, the diseased limb, and this he will be able to do in a degree varying with the previous duration of the affection. While the patient is retained in this position the operator will be able readily to note a rigid cord corresponding to the origin of the adductors, which are invariably the first to shorten.

In fact, this method demonstrates two invariable symptoms of hip joint inflammation, flexion of the hip joint, and curve of the spine, in a greater or lesser degree, so early as the first or second week limiting the normal range of extension, which not only is the patient unable to overcome by his own efforts but which will not yield to the forcible manipulation of the surgeon without the production of

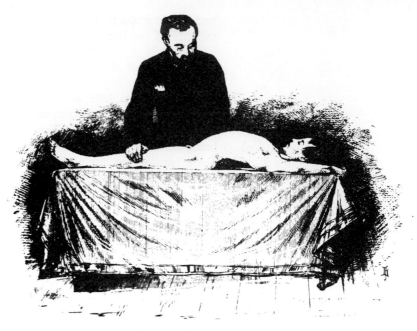

Thomas Hip Flexion Test 1

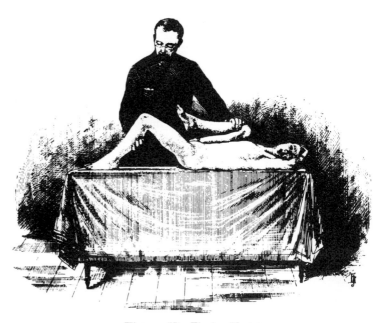

Thomas Hip Flexion Test 2

These wood engravings are taken from photographs of Thomas demonstrating
fixed flexion at the hip joint.

some degree of pain. However on releasing the sound limb from its
flexed position on the chest, the patient may, if not an extreme case,
be able to apparently extend the limb, but a compensatory curve of
the spine is formed.

138

Trendelenburg's Test: Friedrich Trendelenburg, 1844-1924

Born in Berlin, Trendelenburg studied medicine in Glasgow and in Berlin, graduating in 1866. He worked as Assistant to Langenbeck, later filling the Chairs of Surgery at Rostock, Berlin and finally Leipzig.

A prolific writer and leader in practical surgery in many fields, he devised the heroic operation of pulmonary embolectomy, but met with no success. At the age of 80, Kirschner, one of his pupils, demonstrated a successful case to him.

Trendelenburg's Test: 1895

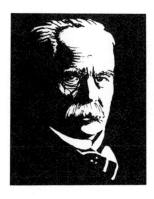

Our knowledge of the anatomical conditions in congenital dislocation of the hip has recently been greatly increased, and has to some extent reached finality as a result of findings at operation. On the other hand the physiological question, as important in practice as it is theoretically interesting, of how the peculiar gait associated with this affection is produced, has not yet been answered; indeed, it has never been properly studied.

Both earlier and more recent authors say only that the cause of the swaying gait is caused by the abnormally mobile femoral head sliding up the ilium when the foot is put down—Dupuytren's "glissement vertical". A few mention the lordosis of the spine as a contributory cause, and all repeat the old comparison of the swinging gait to the waddle of a duck, which, to some extent, describes this type of gait, but does not explain it.

This idea that the abnormal mobility of the head of the femur across the ilium is the cause of the waddling gait is so firmly rooted that the first attempts at surgical treatment did not aim at reduction of the dislocation, but only at fixing the head of the femur to the pelvis (König), and operations of this kind are, even now, performed at times.

If the gait is carefully observed in naked patients it is soon realised that this view is not correct.

A child or, better, an adolescent or adult girl with bilateral congenital dislocation of the hip is told to walk alternately away and towards us. What do we see? Let us look first at the upper part of the body. At every step it swings to and fro, and it does, in fact, fall at each step to the side on which the weight is carried. If the right foot is put down while the left is raised the upper part of the body leans to the right and vice versa. If we call the side of the body with the foot down the standing side and that with the leg swinging the swinging side, the body thus always swings to the standing side. This fact seems to fit the idea that the head of the femur, sliding up when the foot is put down, is the cause of the swaying.

But now let us watch the pelvis. This also sways, in such a way that the right and left sides alternately fall and rise. The pelvis swings on a horizontal axis running from front to back in the sagittal plane at about the level of the first sacral vertebra. But the swing is not in the same direction as the movements of the upper part of the body, but opposite to them. If the right foot is put down, it is not the right anterior superior spine in front and the right buttock at the back which sink, but the left. In other words the pelvis does not, like the upper part of the body, sink on the standing side, but sinks on the swinging side. Now if the swinging movement of the pelvis were caused by the pelvis sliding down past the insufficiently fixed head of the femur the pelvis would sink, like the upper part of the body, on the standing side, and not on the swinging side.

It is precisely the opposing swings of the upper part of the body and the pelvis which is characteristic and peculiar in this gait, as the observer will now realise. He may also remember having seen this gait in only one affection other than bilateral dislocation of the hip, that is, progressive muscular atrophy.

The opposing swings meet between the sacrum and the lumbar spine: this is the pivot of the movements. It looks almost as if a hinge were inserted here, about which the spine moves in relation to the sacrum, and these hinging movements are prompt and full in a way hardly possible in the normal body. The joint has evidently become adapted to the increased demands, and we must expect to find corresponding anatomical changes in older patients. In fact, such changes have already been observed at autopsies, and they will certainly be found more often if they are looked for. In a man of 74 years with bilateral dislocation Dupuytren found at autopsy "a very unusual mobility in the lumbo-sacral joint, so that when the lower extremities and the pelvis were fixed the spine could easily be moved to and fro. Laxity of the intervertebral cartilage was the only recognisable cause of this remarkable mobility"; and Adams found, in a youth of 17 years, with unilateral dislocation that "the intervertebral substance between the last lumbar vertebra and the sacrum was much thicker than usual."

There is another way of demonstrating that the swinging movements are not due to the head of the femur sliding on the ilium. If the patient is told to walk past, or if one walks alongside her and carefully watches the relation of the trochanter to the edge of the pelvis, or feels it with the fingers, it is exceptional to find any distinct rise in the trochanter on putting down the foot; generally this symptom is indefinite, and often it is entirely absent, but the swing still occurs on walking. Movements of up to 2 inches, such as Froriep claims to have seen, do not occur at all in my experience. Even when the patient is lying down and the legs are pulled down, it is very easy to be deceived about the degree of mobility of the head of the femur upwards and downwards.

Moreover, if one compares the gait in various cases of bilateral dislocation, it soon becomes evident that the degree of swinging depends not on the firmer or looser attachment of the head of the femur to the pelvis, but on the position taken by the dislocated head, whether it is fixed or slightly mobile. The higher and further back the head is shifted from the normal place, or in other words, the higher it is and the greater the lordosis, the greater will be the swing. I would mention in passing that the displacement is by no means always proportional to the duration of the affection or to the age of the patient. One sometimes sees adults in whom the trochanters are only two fingers' breadth above the Roser-Nélaton line, and children of four years in whom they have wandered nearly up to the crest of the ilium. The generally made statement that the use of a boot with a raised heel in unilateral dislocation increases the displacement of the head is also, in my opinion, incorrect. At every step the leg must carry the whole weight of the body whether it rests on a high or on a low heel. Children with bilateral dislocation never wear high heels, yet it is particularly in them that a high degree of displacement often occurs very early. Anatomical conditions in the dislocated joint, and not the shape of the shoe, are therefore the deciding factor in the degree of displacement. However, the heel should not be raised enough to compensate wholly for the shortening of the leg for an entirely different reason, namely, to avoid forcing the dislocated joint into adduction, which easily leads to complicating contractures of the adductors.

Now how are these peculiar swinging movements produced? The answer need only deal with the swinging of the pelvis, since it is obvious that the movements of the spine in the opposite direction are only compensatory, and that they perform the task of bringing the centre of gravity, which shifts sideways, back to a point vertically over the standing foot, or, in short, restoring balance.

Let us observe first the gait of a normal person and ascertain in detail how it differs from that in dislocation of the hip. If we make a naked person stand with his back to us behind a plumb line, and make him walk a few steps away from us, we see that the whole body leans alternately a little to the right and left, and always to the side of the foot on the ground. The broader the base of the gait is, the greater the swing, and the more the gait approaches the military slow march, in which each foot is placed as nearly straight in front of the other as possible, the less the swing. The body forms a whole, the pelvis does not swing, but moves evenly forward without swaying. These to and fro movements of the body can easily be fixed photographically without the use of Anschütz's complicated procedure by making the subject examined stand behind a plumb line and raise first one leg and then the other. (I owe Dr. Perthes, Assistant in the Clinic, my special thanks for his help and advice in the sometimes tedious photographic work preliminary to this study). The first glance shows that the swing of the body occurs in order to bring the centre of gravity vertically above the point of support, i.e. the sole of the standing foot. The fact that the pelvis remains horizontal and does not drop on the side of the swinging leg is due to the action of the abductors of the hip joint, the gluteus medius, the gluteus minimus and partly the gluteus maximus. In the standing leg they are stiffly contracted, in the swinging leg they are relaxed. It is easy to ascertain in oneself that this is true in real walking, by putting the hands on the region of the gluteus medius while walking. The alternating play of the muscles can then be felt distinctly.

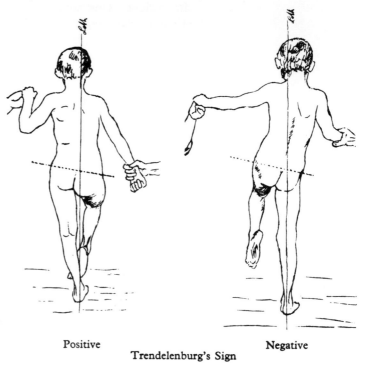

Positive   Trendelenburg's Sign   Negative

Let us compare this with a girl with bilateral dislocation; this girl had to support herself slightly with her hands in order to stand quite still. The difference leaps to the eye. The pelvis hangs down on the swinging side, and the upper part of the body leans far over to the standing side to restore balance.

From what has been said, the cause of the pelvis hanging down can only be that the abductors of the standing leg cannot keep the pelvis horizontal, because, as a result of the anatomical changes resulting from dislocation, they are incapable of holding it. The gluteus medius is reduced to about a third of the normal size, and the direction of its fibres is so altered that it cannot act at all as an abductor. Its anterior part is directed obliquely from the back at the top to the front below, the middle part is horizontal and the posterior part, which alone runs in something like the right direction, is so extremely shortened that its power of traction must be nil. It goes without saying that the action of the gluteus minimus is also completely destroyed, so the whole muscular apparatus providing for abduction of the hips fails.

It is rare to find a child with congenital dislocation who has enough power of abduction to raise the dislocated leg (*in extension*) against gravity when lying on one side.

Since paying attention to this point, I have never seen a child with unilateral dislocation able, when standing on the dislocated leg, to raise the buttock on the other side to the same level as that on the standing side, or even higher, which the same child can easily do when standing on the sound leg, nor have I seen a child with bilateral dislocation able to perform this test standing on either leg. The buttock or the pelvis on the swinging side always hangs down. An intact gluteus medius is essential to develop the relatively great power needed.

Other factors besides the abnormal directions of the fibres and the abnormal shortness of the muscle may contribute to the impairment of its power. When the neck of the femur has disappeared the muscle works on a shorter lever, that is, in more unfavourable conditions, and when the head of the femur remains movable in relation to the ilium the muscle is slackened because its points of insertion come closer together when the foot is put down; it is then too long for the system of levers, and must use part of its power to return to the state in which it can begin to exert an abductor effect. To this extent it must be admitted that the "glissement vertical" contributes indirectly to the swaying gait, though in a quite different way from that hitherto assumed.

If, therefore, the cause of the swaying gait is the absence of active abduction it is easy to understand the similarity of this gait with that in progressive muscular atrophy. In this disease the articular apparatus is intact and the gluteus medius and gluteus minimus have their normal length, but, as in bilateral dislocation, the pelvis is strongly tilted forward as a result of muscular weakness, and there is a corresponding lordosis of the spine. The direction of the fibres of both muscles is therefore more oblique than normally and, even more important, the muscles can only act very incompletely because of the peculiar degeneration. For this reason, the pelvis cannot be held up by the abductors of the hip joint on the standing side and falls towards the swinging side, and the upper part of the body swings in compensation to the other side.

Very defective or entirely absent function of the gluteus medius and gluteus minimus, with the consequent lack of active abduction at the hip, is the cause of the waddling gait in congenital dislocation of the hip.

After treatment the two tests described above—standing on the treated leg and raising the buttock of the other side up to or above the horizontal line and raising the treated leg from the bed while lying on the opposite side—are a good measure of what has been gained by the operation, and the result can also be recorded photographically in this way.

Ortolani's Sign: Marino Ortolani (Contemporary)

Marino Ortolani is Professor of Paediatrics and Child Health, and Director of the Provincial Institute of Infant Welfare at Ferrara. He first described a sign for detecting congenital dislocation of the hip at an early age in 1937—now, a quarter of a century later his test is coming into general use. Why the delay? Partly because he was writing in a little read Italian journal of paediatrics and partly because he presented it as just another sign for examining suspicious hips between the ages of 3 months and 1 year. It was only later that the idea came about that it should be used as a routine in the examination of the new born. This application promises to reduce the number of hips which will require surgery though it will not eliminate the problem.

Ortolani's Sign of Congenital Dislocation of the Hip: 1937

[This extract is taken from his book on C.D.H. published in 1948.]

The sign of "scatto" or snapping, as described by the author, makes the diagnosis a certainty, even in babies. It is probably produced when the head enters or leaves the acetabular cavity, when it jumps over the rim of the acetabulum. This snapping has the same origin as the popping that is usually heard when the hip is reduced during the Paci-Lorenz manoeuvre in the older child under anaesthesia. The "snapping" sign is much more accurate and early than the X-rays or even the arthrogram.

This sign is elicited with the patient lying supine; the hips are flexed to a right angle and internally rotated slightly; the knees are flexed. Holding the knees in the palms of the hands, with the thumbs on the inner aspect of the knees, abduction and external rotation of the hips is carried out. At the same time the fingers press the greater trochanters medially. This manoeuvre, which is quite similar to the manoeuvre of reduction, is not painful and is easily performed when the muscles are relaxed.

Once the "snapping" has been produced, the head of the femur has returned to the acetabular cavity, and the limitation of abduction of the thigh is released.

This sign is due to the fact that from the very first there is an anomalous relationship between the head of the femur and the acetabulum when the leg is flexed on the pelvis. When the thighs are abducted the head comes to jump over the labrum and this gives the sensation of snapping.

The child must be relaxed, otherwise the snapping sign may be missed altogether. This sign may be present even during the child's first month of life.

144

Gauvain's Sign: Sir Henry Gauvain, 1878-1945

The outstanding fact of Gauvain's life is that within two years of leaving medical school he was given charge of a small cripple children's home and from this built a famous orthopaedic hospital. He improved not only the medical care of these children but their social care as well. It is conceivable that his lack of formal training had preserved him from the vapid shibboleths of the time.

He was born in the Channel Isle of Alderney, where his father was Receiver-General. He studied at Cambridge and St. Bartholomew's Hospital, where he held house appointments. In 1908 he became first medical superintendent of the newly opened Lord Mayor Treloar's Cripples Hospital. At first it consisted of a few army huts.

His main interest was bone and joint tuberculosis; he was convinced that surgical attack on the affected joint could not be the right approach as tuberculosis is a generalised disease. "Life in the open air, far from towns, in a dust and germ-free atmosphere, and under the bactericidal and tonic actions of the sun, is the first principle of antibacillary therapeutics." He visited Calvé at Berck-sur-Mer, who had similar ideas. In 1912 he established the first state school in a hospital and the idea soon spread throughout the country. Children were also taught a trade so that when they had recovered they did not find themselves crippled again by unemployment.

He gradually rebuilt the hospital, using a series of wind breaks and sun traps, so that he could get the maximum benefit from the climate.

Perhaps the biggest factor in his success was his happy disposition—he wanted to be friends with everyone. The community thrived on this.

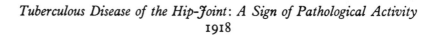

Tuberculous Disease of the Hip-Joint: A Sign of Pathological Activity
1918

In tuberculous disease of the hip-joint, the most constant and most marked evidence of activity is spasm of the muscles about the affected joint. As the disease becomes less acute, spasm becomes increasingly difficult to demonstrate, until eventually it completely disappears. It may last be elicited in the following manner.

DESCRIPTION OF THE SIGN

If the femur, on the affected side, be grasped firmly in the region of the condyles it will be found that the head of the bone may be gently rotated within the acetabulum, either inward or outward, through a varying but often considerable angle. When this movement is checked, but the disease remains active, a further slight sharp rotation is instantly followed by spasmodic muscular contraction, not confined to muscles about the joint but extending to the abdomen and visible in the abdominal muscles, or still more easily demonstrated if the palm of the hand is placed on the abdomen between the iliac spines. Quite a gentle and painless but sharp rotatory movement is sufficient to provoke this reflex spasm of the abdominal muscles. Naturally, it would not be attempted where the disease is obviously active, but in just those cases where doubt exists I have found it a sign of the utmost value.

Confirmatory evidence of activity, as indicated by muscle spasm, may at the same time be demonstrated in the following manner. In a child a finger and thumb of the hand not engaged in grasping the femoral condyles may be applied simultaneously to the two anterior superior iliac spines. During the first rotation of the femur no movement is conveyed to the iliac spines. When, however, rotation has been checked and is sharply but gently continued, exaggerated movement in the same direction is transmitted to the iliac spines.

McMurray's Sign: Thomas Porter McMurray, 1888-1949

McMurray followed Robert Jones at Liverpool, and shared his rooms at 11, Nelson Street—rooms that had been built by Hugh Owen Thomas.

He was born in Belfast, and graduated there in 1910. He then came as a House Surgeon to work for Robert Jones. Later he became lecturer in orthopaedics, and in 1938 occupied the first Chair of Orthopaedics in Liverpool.

McMurray was a man who threw himself into the spirit of things, whether it was relaxing in the country, playing golf or operating. His surgery was dextrous, assured, and very quickly carried out—a meniscus would come out entire in five minutes. It was his dogmatic verbal teaching and training that are remembered, rather than his literary output, which, though important, was not extensive. He wrote a small textbook of orthopaedics in 1937, and an article on Internal Derangements of the Knee, in which he introduced his sign of a torn meniscus. He was one of the originators of osteotomy for arthritis of the hip, an operation which bears his name.

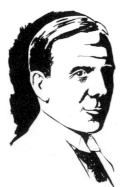

The Diagnosis of Internal Derangements of the Knee: 1928

Lesions of the outer cartilage are, undoubtedly, much more difficult of diagnosis than those of the inner cartilage, especially in those cases in which the definite snap, so typical of these lesions, is not present, and lesions of the posterior end of the internal cartilage give a much less definite train of symptoms than those of the anterior end, and for these cases I have found an accessory method of diagnosis of the greatest help.

In using this method the knee should be flexed completely, so that the heel rests on the buttock or as near this point as possible: the ankle is then grasped in the right hand, and the joint controlled by the left hand with the thumb and fore-finger firmly grasping it on either side at the level of the joint to its posterior aspect, and behind the external and internal lateral ligaments respectively. The ankle is now twisted by the right hand, so that the knee is rotated inwards and outwards to its fullest extent, and if a lesion of the external cartilage or of the posterior portion of the internal cartilage is present a definite click can be felt under the finger or thumb of the left hand. Examination of an abnormally lax knee-joint in which there is no lesion of the internal or external cartilages may give a sensation which might at first be mistaken for this click, but in such a case the click is not definite, and there is never the peculiar sliding or gliding of the femur over an apparent obstacle which is so typically present when there has been an injury to the external cartilage or posterior portion of the internal.

As an aid in the diagnosis of doubtful knee-joint lesions this method of examination has been of the greatest help to me, because it is applicable in just those cases which are otherwise so difficult, and in which a correct diagnosis is essential. It is by this means that I have been able to diagnose correctly on many occasions an injury to the posterior end of the semilunar cartilage, which at operation on first opening of the joint appeared to be perfectly normal. This method is inapplicable to lesions of the anterior end of the internal semilunar cartilage, but this, fortunately, is of little moment, because diagnosis here is usually comparatively easy, and should give rise to little trouble if sufficient care is exercised.

Froment's Sign: Jules Froment, 1878-1946

Jules Froment was Professor of Medicine at Lyons, and devoted his life to neurology, combining diligent observation, a philosophical approach and debating skill.

Graduating in 1906 with a thesis on disease of the heart in thyrotoxicosis, he remained at Lyons until the Great War. After a year at the front, he joined a nerve injuries unit at Rennes, and later was at Paris with Babinski. During this time he evolved a series of tests for nerve dysfunction, the best known being his sign of ulnar nerve weakness; another was loss of the hollow of the anatomical snuff box in radial nerve injury.

After the war he ran a Red Cross Hospital in Lyons, and the encephalitis epidemic of 1918-1922 provided another intellectual challenge. In 1926 he nearly died as a result of being severely injured by one of his patients.

Froment pointed out the difference between a pinch grip and grasping, both of which are impaired by a low ulnar nerve palsy due to weakness of adductor pollicis. He introduced the following test to show this. Today it is used to assess flexor pollicis brevis.

Froment's Signe du Pouce: 1915

In order to demonstrate the disorder of the grip it is sufficient for the patient to take hold of any object between the thumb and other fingers. Two features may be observed: first, the weakness of the grip, and secondly the abnormal position of the thumb, although, while at rest, nothing would lead one to suspect it.

It is when a thin object is gripped that the faulty position of the thumb is most clearly evident. In practice, we hold out a folded newspaper to the patient; he is asked to pull it hard with the strong hand and then with the affected hand, while we pull it fairly firmly away. This is what is observed: on the healthy side the thumb is in contact with the object gripped all the way along—the distal phalanx is extended or only slightly flexed. On the paralysed side the thumb resembles a flying buttress, the distal phalanx is markedly flexed and no matter what force is used it only holds the object by the very tip of the pulp. Very often there is a gap between the thumb and the newspaper, or, to be more exact, between the thumb and the side of the palm. (It is necessary to pull hard: the grip with the fixed thumb is only pathological when the grip is forcible).

This asymmetric attitude between the thumbs appears very clearly when the patient, taking the newspaper in both hands, pulls with different strength at both ends. This can clearly be seen in the photograph.

Tinel's Sign: Jules Tinel, 1879-1952

Tinel was a French neurologist who wrote an excellent book on the effects of nerve injuries during the First World War, and from it one may judge how times have changed, for nerve suture is hardly mentioned. He had a research interest in the autonomic system, producing a thick volume on the subject; he was noted for the ingenuity of his apparatus, which was often constructed of Meccano.

He was born in Rouen, the fifth in a line of distinguished doctors. His father was Professor of Anatomy at Rouen. Tinel studied in Paris. It was when he was mobilised for the war that he found himself in a neurological unit and was able to study the long term effects of severe nerve injury. He gave the first account of paroxysmal hypertension due to phaeochromocytoma.

During the Second World War he had to leave the Hospital; his family were interned, and one son executed by the Gestapo because they had helped run an escape route.

148

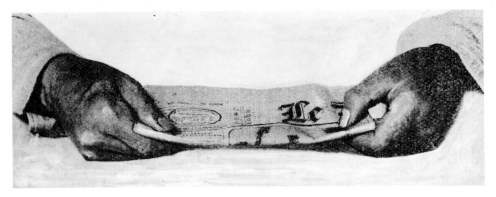

Froment's Sign

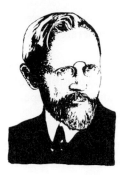

Tinel's Sign: 1917

Formication provoked by pressure.—When compression or percussion is lightly applied to the injured nerve trunk, we often find, in the cutaneous region of the nerve, a creeping sensation usually compared by the patient to that caused by electricity.

Formication in the nerve is a very important sign, for it indicates the presence of young axis-cylinders in process of regeneration.

This formication is quite distinct from the pain on pressure, which exists in nerve irritations. Tenderness, indicating irritation of the axis-cylinders and not their regeneration, is almost always local, perceived at the very spot where the nerve is compressed, or at least magnified at this spot; it always co-exists with the pain in the muscular bellies under pressure, which are, very often, more tender than the nerve.

Formication of regeneration, on the other hand, is but little or not at all perceived at the spot compressed, but is felt almost entirely in the cutaneous distribution of the nerve; the neighbouring muscles are not tender.

As a rule, it appears only about the fourth or sixth week after the wound. It enables us to ascertain the existence of this regeneration and to follow its progress.

If it remains fixed and limited to one spot for several consecutive weeks or months, this is because the regenerating axis-cylinders have encountered an insurmountable obstacle and are forced together at that place as a more or less bulky neuroma.

The fixity of formication on a level with the lesion, and the complete absence of formication below the lesion, would almost warrant our affirming the complete interruption of the nerve and the impossibility of spontaneous regeneration.

If, on the other hand, the regenerated axis-cylinders can overcome the obstacle and make their way into the peripheral segment of the nerve, we see a progressive migration of the formication so provoked. Pressure on the nerve below the wound produces this sensation, and from week to week it may be encountered at a spot farther removed from the nerve lesion. The presence of formication provoked by pressure below the nerve lesion warrants our affirming that there is more or less complete regeneration.

The site at which formication can be demonstrated moves along the course of the nerve at the same pace as the axis-cylinders advance; at the same time that it extends progressively towards the periphery it disappears at the level of the lesion.

The "formication sign" is thus of supreme importance, since it enables us to see whether the nerve is interrupted, or is in course of regeneration; whether a nerve suture has succeeded or failed, or whether regeneration is rapid and satisfactory, or reduced to a few significant fibres.

Formication lasts a tolerably long time; appearing about the fourth week, it persists during the entire regeneration, i.e., for eight, ten, twelve months or more, gradually drawing nearer the extremity of the limb. It ceases only when the regenerated axis-cylinders have almost regained their adult stage.

Formication, however, may be absent, both at the level of the lesion and below it; this absence is an unfavourable prognostic point; it shows that nerve regeneration is taking place imperfectly, mainly because of general disturbances of nutrition.

He discusses examination of the peripheral nerves and points out that in neuralgia there may be nerve tenderness; after section there is formication, or tingling distally, and neuromata are palpable.

The Lasègue Sign

The remarkable feature of this sign is that it was never described by Lasègue —the 'universal specialist'. In 1864 Lasègue wrote 'Thoughts of Sciatica' and since then most authors have been happy to imagine that this includes a description of the sign. This error has been copied from one learned book to another. Lasègue in fact described two cases of sciatica observing that weight bearing and flexing both hip and knee together aggravated the pain.

His pupil Forst described the sign in a doctoral thesis in 1881, and wrote that his attention was attracted to it by his teacher, sponsor, and President of the University examiners—Lasègue. Forst considered that the sign depended on the sciatic nerve becoming compressed by the hamstrings.

However, in the year before Forst went into print a Yugoslavian physician, Laza K. Lazarevic, had described the sign in the *Serbian Archives*. Lazarevic based his observations on six patients and realised that the sciatic nerve could be stretched by straight leg raising. He mentioned two other ways of eliciting the sign: by attempted toe touching, or alternatively by instructing the patient to sit up in bed with his knees extended. Due to the lack of popularity of this last technique it is a useful way of detecting a malingerer.

In 1884 de Beurmann studied the mechanism of the sign; he removed the sciatic nerve from a cadaver, replacing it by a piece of rubber tubing. On straight leg raising the tube elongated by 8 cm.

There seems little point in immortalising the name of Lasègue in this connection. Lazarevic or Forst would prove no more popular with medical secretaries—perhaps it should be called the sciatic stretch test.

Sciatic Stretch Test: J. J. Forst, 1881

We do not intend to make a complete study of sciatica but will limit ourselves to study, in particular, one clinical sign of very great value from the point of view of diagnosis. In spite of all that has been written on sciatica, we have been unable to find any mention of the symptom that we are about to discuss. Professor Lasègue attracted my attention to this sign.

What then is this sign?

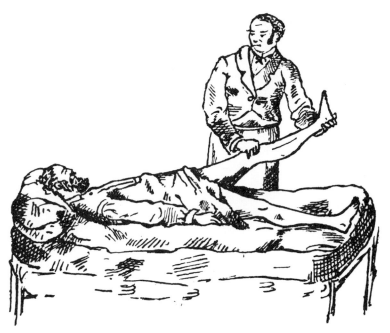

Sciatic Stretch Test demonstrated by J. J. Forst.

We place the patient on the bed lying on his back; in this position we take the foot of the affected leg in one hand as shown in Figure, and place the other hand on the knee of the same leg; having done this, we flex the thigh on the pelvis, keeping the leg extended; it is only necessary to lift the limb a few inches for the patient to experience acute pain at the level of the sciatic notch just at the emergence of the nerve. We replace the limb on the bed, and proceed with another manoeuvre, which gives further verification of the sign that we have mentioned.

We have just seen that the patient experiences acute pain when the thigh is flexed on the pelvis while the leg is held in extension. If we now flex the leg at the knee, we are able to flex the thigh at the hip without causing the patient any painful feeling.

Forst reasons that the pain is produced by the muscles at the back of the thigh becoming tense when the straight leg raising test is performed. These muscles compress the sciatic nerve. When the knee is flexed the relaxed muscles do not compress the nerve and the manoeuvre is painless.

PART FIVE

TREATMENT

The object of treatment is the restoration of complete function with least risk and inconvenience to the patient and with least anxiety to the surgeon.

Robert Jones, 1913.

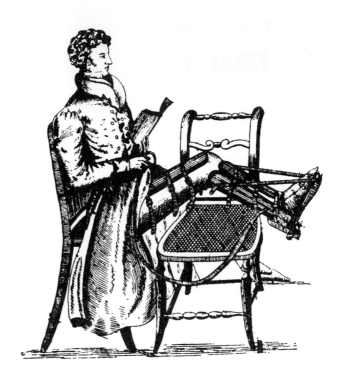

1 SPLINTS AND APPARATUS

A broken bone cannot be too soon put to rights.

Percivall Pott.

Bandaging should be done quickly, without pain, with ease and with elegance.

Hippocrates.

Positions for Splinting Limbs:

Paré, in the sixteenth century, was one of the first to draw attention to the ill effects resulting from splinting limbs, or allowing them to remain, in a bad position. By choice, limbs should be splinted in a functional position.

Vicious posture increases ill symptoms.
When the wound is in the wrist or joints of the fingers either internally or externally, the hand must be kept half shut continually moving a ball therein. For if the fingers be held straight stretched

forth, after it is cicatrized, they will be unapt to take up or hold anything, which is their proper faculty. But if after it is healed it remains half shut, no great inconvenience will follow thereon: for so may he use his hand diverse ways to his sword, pike, bridle, or in anything else.

Paré suggested that other parts should be splinted as follows:

Shoulder — bolster placed in the axilla
Elbow — midway between the extremes of flexion and extension
Knee — extended
Hip — extended

Function of Splints:

The true and proper use of splints is, to preserve steadiness in the whole limb, without compressing the fracture at all. By the former they become very assistant to the curative intention; by the latter they are very capable of causing pain and other inconveniences; at the same time that they cannot, in the nature of things, contribute to the steadiness of the limb.

In order to be of any real use at all, splints should, in the case of a broken leg, reach above the knee and below the ankle.

By this they become really serviceable; but a short splint, which only extends a little above and a little below the fracture, and does not take in the two joints, is an absurdity; and, what is worse, it is a mischievous absurdity.

Pott, 1769.

Plaster of Paris Bandages

In the days of Hippocrates, bandages that set hard were used for nasal fractures. Initially, wheat glues, and later, wax and resins were used. Rhazes, an Arabian physician of the ninth century, wrote: "But if thou make thine apparatus with lime and white of egg, it will be much handsomer and will not need to be removed until the healing is complete."

In the eighteenth century, Cheselden in England was a keen advocate of egg-white bandages for fractures and the correction of club feet, but in Arabia plaster was used. Mr. Eton, the British Consul in Bassora, wrote in 1798:-

I saw in the Eastern parts of the Empire a method of setting bones practised, which appears to be worthy of the attention of surgeons in Europe. It is by enclosing the broken limb, after the bones are put in their places, in a case of plaster of Paris (gypsum) which takes exactly the form of the limb, without any pressure, and in a few minutes the mass is solid and strong. . . . This substance may be easily cut with a knife, and removed, and replaced with another. If when the swelling subsides the cavity is too large for the limb, a hole or holes being left, liquid gypsum plaster may be poured in, which will perfectly fill up the void, and exactly fit the limb. A hole may be made at first by placing an oiled cork or bit of wood against any part where it is required, and when the plaster is set, it is to be removed. There is nothing in gypsum injurious, if it be free from lime; it will soon become very dry and light, and the limb may be bathed with spirits, which will penetrate through the covering. I saw a case of a most terrible compound fracture of the leg and thigh, by the fall of a cannon, cured in this manner. The person was seated on the ground, and the plaster case extended from below the heel to the upper part of this thigh, whence a bandage, fastened into the plaster, went round his body.

In India, too, similar methods were used. Sir George Ballingall wrote in *Outline of Military Surgery* in 1852:-

> The practice of enveloping fractured limbs in splints and bandages, without undoing them, for weeks together, is akin to that followed by the natives of India of enclosing fractured limbs in moulds of clay. Of the successful result of this practice I remember a remarkable instance in the case of a little boy who was brought into my tent one morning, having been run over by a waggon on the line of march, and having sustained a severe compound fracture of the leg. I was preparing to amputate this boy's limb when the parents came in and carried him away to a potter in an adjoining village, who enveloped the leg in clay, and I believe finally cured the patient.

In Europe Hubenthal seems to have used plaster of Paris in 1816; it was mixed with ground up blotting paper. Twelve years later Koyle and Kluge introduced a plaster box to the Charité Hospital, Berlin. The injured limb was laid in a wooden box into which plaster was poured. But while these developments were going on, egg white remained the favourite bonding agent. Gentin, Senior Medical Officer of the Belgian Army, inaugurated a period of starch bandages in 1834 and realised that it was better if patients with fractures of the leg could be ambulatory.

Another Army surgeon—Mathysen, in the Dutch Army—introduced plaster bandages in 1852. The technique was popularised by its extensive use in the Crimean War. In America, Samuel St. John of New York was a strong advocate of plaster because, he taught, the splint should be fitted to the limb, and not the limb to the splint. He introduced the padding of plasters with cotton wadding and, like Mathysen, split the plaster while wet.

But voices were raised against plaster immobilisation of fractures—Hugh Owen Thomas wrote that "it did not allow frequent inspection, was much labour at first, and little afterwards, and provided no opportunity for the display of skill". He thought that compression and covering up an injured limb reduced its vitality. A splint allowed the position to be improved as the fracture softened. Fixation of fractured bones, Thomas considered, "merely favours their early and normal repair, and tends to discourage the formation of supplementary matter". About the same time, a man with ideas diametrically opposed to Thomas, Lucas Champonnière was questioning the tenets of fracture treatment. He was concerned with movement after the fracture had healed. "The return of the limb to the maximum possible muscular strength, and the maximum joint mobility is a hundred times more important than the exact form of the skeleton." Callus formation was encouraged by regulated movement which kept the joints moving. Further, if the limb were left free, the bone remained strong and was less likely to refracture.

While it was the Crimean War that spread the word about plaster fixation, it was the First World War, when radiology was used for the first time on a large scale for the treatment of fractures, that standardised the use of plaster.

Antonius Mathysen, 1805-1878

Mathysen was born in Brudel, a small village in N. Brabant, Holland, of a medical family, and trained as a military surgeon at Brussels and Utrecht. In 1831 he was involved in a 10-day campaign in Belgium and was decorated.

Mathysen wrote a short paper on plaster splints in 1852 and a monograph in 1854. The idea caught on rapidly—in 1858 he devised plaster shears and was widely honoured for his inventiveness. A monument was erected in 1948 at Brudel to commemorate him and his portrait appeared on a Dutch stamp.

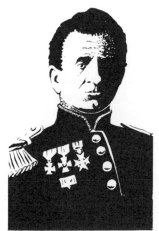

The Invention of Plaster Appliances: Mathysen, 1852

At the end of 1851, when I was stationed at Harlem (N. Holland), I made my first attempt to use plaster for surgical treatment. The bandages which I made at that time consisted of a layer of dry plaster in powder form spread evenly between two compresses. The wounded limb was placed on this; the bandage was then well wetted and wound around the limb. In this way the wounded limb was given a solid shell; however, when one wanted to strip off this casing to examine the injured parts, the bed of plaster broke, and the bandage lost its shape and strength.

Soon I succeeded in introducing an improved modification to this poultice-like bandage. Immediately after having wet the bandage, I marked out a groove along it, parallel to the limb, using the edge of a spatula; in this way the plaster could be hinged and one could even separate the slabs without running the risk of breaking or damaging the plaster.

As I realised that my methods had resulted in success I continued my experiments assiduously for, although the groove allowed the bandage to be removed fairly easily, it was still far from what it should be to compete with other methods of treatment; it was too heavy and was not firm enough.

To overcome these problems, I looked for a substance which could be mixed with the plaster to give it more firmness, render it less easily breakable and thus obtain a strong appliance. However, my search proved fruitless.

Then I struck upon the idea of spreading the plaster in thin layers between three or four compresses and rubbing it into the closely woven weft of the pieces of material. The result was just what I wanted: the appliances made from these plastered pieces of material were light, firm, and elastic, and thus I realised my aim.

Soon I also tried using plaster with pieces of cotton and partly worn linen which worked perfectly—in this way I obtained cotton-plaster. From the original large sheet I cut off pieces in various sized strips, with which I very easily made various types of bandage. These bandages satisfied me on all counts, and I can confidently attribute them with the following properties and advantages:-

(1) *Simplicity*: To make up plaster bandages one only needs some cotton or woollen material, some plaster, and water, and one can dispense with splints and other similar things.

(2) *Easy Application*: The strips of bandage can be put on in the easiest way: one winds the plastered pieces around the affected part like ordinary bandages; they shape themselves, so to speak, and one immediately obtains a solid shell which encases the affected part exactly.

(3) *Instant Setting*: This is a quality which no other appliance possesses, and this gives a particular advantage to plaster bandage. To justify this statement, one has only to consider fracture cases which involve fretful children, agitated or delirious patients, and above all, injuries on the battlefield. This instant setting property of plaster would allow the evacuation of battlefield casualties by any means of transport, without exposing them to the appalling dangers and suffering with which they are threatened today.

(4) Plaster bandages can be applied *without assistance*.

(5) Plaster bandages can be applied *in a few minutes*.

(6) *Complete fixation*: This bandage can be made so firm that it resists heavy knocks.

(7) *Removability*: The plaster appliance can be applied straight away as a bivalve. One can easily change the fixed bandage into a removable one, by cutting with large scissors.

(8) It has *exact retention*, because the plaster bandage encases the parts with the same strength all over; the parts rest on as wide a surface as possible—for this reason the injured part is well supported and does not become tired.

(9) The plaster bandage maintains *extension and counter-extension* from the time of application. Because of this one does not need any other temporary appliances, as one does with other fixed apparatus.

(10) *Porosity*: This property allows cutaneous perspiration to evaporate through the plaster shell, and also allows any other fluid

secreted beneath the bandage to come through the plaster and thus give warning of unexpected complications.

(11) The plaster appliance *resists all types of liquid action*: neither urine, pus nor water harm its firmness or strength in any way.

(12) Plaster can be *easily removed*: to do so, one wets the bandage with water and unrolls it like an ordinary bandage—in a few minutes one can remove or re-apply the plaster bandage.

(13) *Price*: no other appliance is as cheap.

(14) *Appearance*: the plaster appliance excels in its regular and beautiful appearance.

From all the properties that I have just mentioned one can conclude a priori that not only can these bandages be applied in cases of fractures of the limbs and trunk, but also in cases of those infirmities known as orthopaedic maladies, and in general in all cases in which M. Seutin has used his starch bandages; also, this technique has the advantage that dressings can be greatly simplified: splints, cradles, etc., can be abandoned; there is also the advantage of having fewer objects to carry about, which is of the greatest importance, particularly in battlefield surgery.

It is obvious that one could also use these bandages very advantageously in *veterinary surgery*.

The Thomas Splint: Hugh Owen Thomas

Robert Jones' Views on Thomas Splints: 1925

The Great War afforded the most convincing proof of the mishandling of complicated, and even of simple, fractures. Fractures of the femur serve as a notable example. The splint with which we are all so familiar, invented by Thomas, was barely known, and yet it was the type of splint which ultimately saved the situation. In 1916 the mortality from these fractures amounted to 80 per cent., a large proportion of the deaths occurring on their way to or at Casualty Clearing Stations. Later, when the Thomas Splint was applied almost exclusively, and as near to the firing line as possible the mortality in 1918 was reduced to 20 per cent.

(It is ironic that on one of the few occasions Hugh Owen Thomas left his practice, he went to offer this splint to the French Army in the eighteen seventies, and that it was refused.)

The Knee Appliance: Hugh Owen Thomas, 1875

The upper crescent is formed of an iron ring three-eighths of an inch thick, varying according to the age and weight of the patient; the ring is nearly ovoid in shape and is covered with boiler felt and basil leather; from its upper and lower portions two iron rods pass down to the lower end of the machine, where may be noticed a small staple for retention purposes, only used for the reduction of flexion.

The ovoid ring should join the inner stem, forming an angle of 55 degrees, which when correctly padded becomes reduced to 45 degrees. This arrangement of the splint will be the most acceptable for wearing. The staple can be cut off at a subsequent stage and replaced by a patten, which is welded on in its place, for the use of the patient in locomotion.

This was designed for the treatment of tuberculous knees in order to achieve "prolonged uninterrupted and enforced rest" in the extended position so that the infection could settle and leave an undeformed joint. He also used it for femoral shaft fractures, and to mobilise amputations before a prosthesis could be fitted. The basic splint had several variations. He put wheels on the lower end to make it more comfortable in bed rather than sling it up. The lower end had a patten for walking, and he developed one with the ring in two halves (inner and outer) for use when the knee was very swollen.

Traction

Since the earliest days traction has been used to reduce dislocations. Hippocrates used his heel, ladders, poles, and a sort of rack known as the scamnum of Hippocrates. His successors vied with one another to produce ever more fearsome equipment with more pulleys, longer levers, and stronger ropes. These were for short sharp pulls. This sort of equipment was quite unsuited for prolonged traction as it damaged the skin and impaired the circulation. Anaesthesia has largely abolished the need for brute force; there are only a few machines in current use, such as Hawley's table and Bohler's frame for tibial fractures, which remind us of those rack and pinion days.

It is not surprising that continuous traction is of recent origin. In the past, unreduced simple fractures and circumferential bandages used to produce their toll of ulcers, gangrene, and erysipelas, without adding the hazard of badly applied continuous traction. A method of applying continuous traction without these complications proved difficult to find. Fractures of the femur were the first to be treated by continuous traction as the undamaged shin provided some sort of purchase. In the eighteenth century several surgeons, such as Pott and Petit, began to use inclined planes. They had the first realisation that gravity could be used to maintain the position. Much later, in 1839, John Haddy James of Exeter (1788-1869) described continuous traction using a weight suspended over a pulley. He bandaged the leg to a wooden splint that rested on rollers; a string from the splint passed over a pulley to a weight. As he did not tip the bed, the patient was fixed to the headboard by a harness, to prevent him being pulled out of bed feet first by the weight.

Josse, of Amiens, had solved the problem differently two years before. He lashed the patient's foot to the end of the bed, which was raised.

It was some 26 years before the two ideas were amalgamated.

Straight leg traction was popularised in the American Civil War. At the beginning of this war, in 1860, Gurdon Buck described a simple form of traction, easily applied in wartime conditions. His description follows later, from which it will be seen that the meaning of Buck's traction was changed through the years.

It was another war, the Balkan war, that saw the introduction, by a Dutch ambulance unit, of the Balkan beam in 1903. About this time the standard of conservative treatment received a stimulus to improve; X-rays and internal fixation were becoming available. A poor position was less easily tolerated and the search began for more sophisticated forms of traction. Codivilla tried applying traction to a below knee plaster, but found that it produced skin necrosis. Skeletal traction was introduced. It had its antecedents in the ice tongs that Malgaine used to hold a fractured patella together, more than 50 years before. Martin Kirschner (1879-1942), a surgeon at Heidelberg, used thin wires in 1909; he inserted them at first both above and below the fracture line and, with the aid of a distraction apparatus, prevented overlapping. Fritz Steinmann (1872-1932), a surgeon at Berne, introduced thicker pins and stirrups in 1911. He introduced the sites at which this form of traction is applied—femoral condyle, tibial tubercle and calcaneum.

At its inception opponents to skeletal traction maintained that it was a "compromise between inefficient closed operation and a hazardous open operation".

Buck's Traction: Gurdon Buck, 1807-1877

Buck was a general surgeon in New York. He described a form of extension for fractures of the femoral shaft just before the American Civil War. It proved popular in the war and preserved his name for posterity.

Genealogists have established that the Gurdon family came to England with William the Conqueror, and another stem came to America with the Pilgrim Fathers. His father ran a shipping business in New York. Gurdon studied medicine, and graduated in 1830. After a period as a House Physician at New York Hospital, he came to Europe to study surgery, spending two years visiting Paris, Vienna and Berlin.

In 1837 he was visiting surgeon to the New York Hospital. His particular field of interest was plastic surgery—the Civil War left an aftermath of facial injuries which he repaired with rotation and pedicle flaps; secondary defects were left to heal by themselves. A year before he died, he published a classic, entitled *Reparative Surgery* which is filled with striking illustrations. In addition he was a good anatomist, describing Buck's fascia of the perineum.

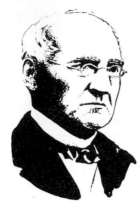

Buck's Extension: 1860

Dr. Gurdon Buck read an interesting paper upon a new treatment for fractures of the femur, of which the following is an abstract:-

The appliances to the limb itself for the purpose of making extension are the same as have been in use in our hospitals for several years past, and are as follows:- A roller bandage is commenced at the toes in the usual way, and continued to the ankles, where it is temporarily arrested. A band of adhesive plaster two and a half to three inches broad, and long enough to allow the middle of it to form a loop below the sole of the foot, and the ends to extend above the condyles of the femur, is then applied on either side, in immediate contact with the limb, from the ankle upwards. Over this the bandage is continued as high up as the plaster. A thin block of wood of the width of the plaster, and long enough to prevent pressure over the ankle, is inserted into the loop, and serves for the attachment of the extending cord, which is fastened to an elastic rubber band (such as is used for door springs) that passes round the block. By this arrangement *elasticity* is combined with the extension. The limb is now prepared to be put under extension. The arrangement for the pulley is very simple. A strip of inch board three inches wide is fastened upright to the foot of the bedstead, and perforated at the height of four or five inches above the level of the mattress. Through this hole the extending cord is to be passed, and on the further side of the strap a screw pulley should be inserted at the proper level over which the cord, with the weight attached, is to play. The foot-board of the bedstead, if there is one, may be perforated at the proper level, and the screw pulley inserted in the further side of it, so as to answer equally well. To allow the application of lotions to the thigh during the first few days of treatment, the ends of the adhesive bands should stop short at the condyles of the femur, and be turned down. They may afterwards be replaced upon the thigh and the bandages continued over them, preparatory to the application of the coaptation splints, which should be added at this stage of the treatment. The coaptation splints, which may be of the ordinary sort, should be secured by those elastic bands, like suspender webbing fitted with buckles; these have the advantage of keeping up uniform concentric pressure as the limb diminishes from the subsidence of swelling. Counter-extension must be maintained by the usual perineum band lengthened out in the direction of the long axis of the body, and fastened to the head of the bedstead. India rubber tubing of three-quarters of an inch calibre, stuffed with a skein of cotton lamp wick, makes an excellent perineum strap. A piece of two feet long with a ring fastened at each end answers this purpose admirably. A thin wedge-shaped hair cushion, to raise the heel above the mattress, and a bag filled with bran or sand to place on the outside of the foot to prevent rotation outwards, complete the appliances requisite to carry out this method of treatment. There need be no delay in its application. The sooner after the occurrence of the injury, the limb is put up, the better. The contraction of the muscles is thus antagonised from the outset, and the rough ends of the fragments are prevented from fretting the soft parts.

The author then gave twenty-one cases in detail where this treatment was employed; and the results, as shown by *actual measurement*, are equal to any that have hitherto been obtained. Dr. Buck claims for the apparatus the following advantages:-

I. It maintains *uninterrupted* and *efficient extension* without producing intolerable pain, excoriations, sloughing, and tedious sores.

II. It diminishes very materially the suffering of the patient and the irksomeness of long confinement to one position. There is no inconvenience attending the evacuation of the bowels.

III. It is cheap and easy of application.

IV. It is not liable to become deranged, thus rendering it unnecessary for as frequent visits on the part of the surgeon as when the ordinary apparatus is applied. The author considers it very necessary to apply coaptation splints, for reasons already given.

Russell Traction: Robert Hamilton Russell, 1860-1933

Russell was born in Kent and studied under Lister, and was his House Surgeon. He emigrated to Melbourne in 1890. He brought antiseptic surgery with him and did much to establish a high standard of general surgery in Australia. In particular he founded the College of Surgeons of Australasia and was its first Director-General.

He is remembered for devising a very useful system of traction; though now used to relieve the painful spasm of an irritable hip from any cause it was designed for something different. Percivall Pott used to teach that the deformity of long bone fractures was maintained by muscle pull and that the muscles must be relaxed for reduction to be stable. Russell had the same approach—his traction was designed to circumvent undesirable muscle spasm in fractures of the femur. It is not much used today as it requires constant vigilance.

In the outback he sustained a Colles' fracture and as there was no medical help near he promptly reduced it himself and continued to treat it.

He was killed in a motor accident.

Fracture of the Femur: A Clinical Study, 1924

Let us suppose a patient with fracture of the middle of the femoral shaft just admitted to hospital.

The Thigh is Shortened. Why?—The shortening is caused by the tonic contraction of certain long muscles that are attached above to the pelvic bone, and traverse the entire length of the thigh to be

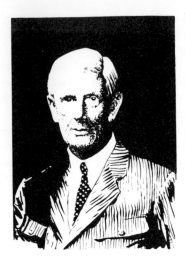

inserted into the tibia and fibula. Of these there are two opposing sets, consisting (in the main) of the hamstrings and the rectus femoris.

The numerous muscles that are attached to the femur itself play little if any part in the production of shortening.

Muscular *tone* (which must always be carefully distinguished in our minds from muscular *action*) is a physiological property of living muscle, which for practical purposes causes the muscles to behave like rubber bands slightly stretched. Their correct length is maintained by the length of the femur, and as soon as the femur is broken they shorten and produce over-riding of the fragments. Here the analogy ends, for rubber once released from its tension will have no further power of contraction, whereas the tonic shortening of the muscles will be progressive. Hence the excessive shortening, amounting to three or four inches, that almost invariably complicates an ununited fracture of the femur.

Our first aim, then, will be to pull out these muscles to their correct length; and when we have accomplished this we may be sure that every other structure in the thigh will be in its correct position, including the fragments.

What must we Pull upon?—Clearly the tibia and fibula, seeing that the muscles are attached to them. We are going to use strappings and bandages for the extension, and we shall accordingly not carry them above the knee, for reasons that are obvious. I think that the practice, which seems universal, of carrying the strapping up the thigh indicates some confusion in our mental picture of the object to be attained. Anxiety as regards the ligaments of the knee seems also to be felt; but this is quite needless, for the ligaments of the knee, being attached to a fragment, cannot be subjected to stretching. The whole of the extending force will fall on the muscles, none at all on the ligaments; to convince ourselves of this we only have to reflect that if the muscles were severed at the seat of fracture the limb would drop off.

How must we Pull upon the Tibia and Fibula?—If we merely attach a weight to the leg to pull out the thigh muscles, it is obvious that the leg and thigh will have to be in a straight line, or the thigh muscles cannot be extended. But this will never do; for one among several reasons, it would be intolerably uncomfortable; and perfect comfort, as we shall see, is the first essential requirement in any appliance for the treatment of a fracture. We must have the knee slightly bent; but the bending of the knee is incompatible with the necessary pull on the thigh muscles that are attached to the tibia and fibula.

In a difficulty of this kind I always advise my students to do this. First take hold of the fractured limb with both hands and bring it into perfect position. Holding it thus, study carefully the position and *direction* of the forces you are applying. Then see if you can devise some plan of incorporating similar forces in an apparatus of some kind. In the case of the fractured femur, how does the surgeon

164

manipulate it in order to draw out the thigh muscles? He will do it in the following way. Standing by the side of the bed he passes the left hand under the knee; the right hand grasps the leg above the ankle. Now he gradually exerts a little power, the right hand pulling horizontally towards the foot of the bed, the left hand up towards the ceiling mostly, but with a slight inclination footwards also. The direction of the forces being exerted by the surgeon's hands are indicated by the arrows in the picture. The limb will not come out to its proper length all at once, but the patient will feel more comfortable, and will instinctively know that his limb is being skilfully and properly handled.

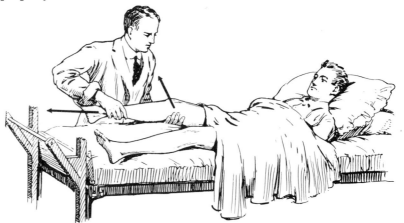

The Theory of Hamilton Russell Traction

The surgeon now reasons thus: I am sure that this is the right way to get the thigh out to its proper length if only the thigh muscles were quiescent; but they are not, owing to the patient's apprehension and fever. Were I able to stand here doing this for a few hours or until he sleeps, then there would be no difficulty; but obviously that is not possible. I must then devise some means of doing what I am now doing; something that will not tire, that will make the limb absolutely comfortable; and in that way favour the return of mental quietude.

The Apparatus.—The arrangement shown in figure was evolved in the way just described—a sling beneath the knee corresponding to the surgeon's left hand and horizontal traction on the leg corresponding to the surgeon's right hand. The arrangement provides that the pull on the leg shall be nominally double the upward lift at the knee, although actually somewhat modified by friction between pulleys and cord.

Application of the Apparatus.—Usually an anaesthetic is not required; children have been known to sleep through the whole procedure.

1. The leg having been prepared in the ordinary way is fitted with a spreader or stirrup close to the sole of the foot by a method similar to that used in 'Buck's extension', but with two important

differences: (a) The strapping is not carried above the knee; (b) The spreader is provided with a pulley; its essential feature is that it must be long enough (5 in.) to deflect the strapping sufficiently to protect the malleoli from pressure. A light bandage over all from the roots of the toes to the knee, and the leg is ready.

2. The placing of the pulleys. First, pulley A is tied to the over-head bar in such a position that a vertical dropped from it shall meet the leg well below the knee. Pulleys B and D are to be attached separately to the bar beyond the foot of the bed; pulley C is that attached to the spreader.

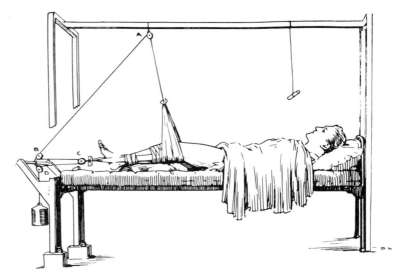

Hamilton Russell Traction

3. The knee-sling is now passed beneath the knee, which all this time has been lying comfortably on a pillow. The sling should be broad and soft; a soft rough towel suitably folded answers well. The ends of the sling are now securely tied together with the cord, which is then passed through the pulleys in the following order: (a) Up to pulley A; (b) To pulley B beyond the bed; (c) To pulley C on the spreader; (d) To pulley D (companion to B).

4. The surgeon now stands at the foot of the bed and slowly tightens up everything, and then the weight is attached. He next takes a soft pillow and adjusts it comfortably beneath the thigh to prevent gravitational sagging at the seat of fracture. Care must be taken that the pillow is really soft; a common fault is to have too hard and tightly-stuffed a pillow for this purpose. Next he looks to the heel; it must not be touching the bed, and he arranged another soft pillow beneath the leg and tendo Achillis to prevent it from doing so. And now the patient will be absolutely comfortable, and rest of both mind and body (including thigh muscles) will come to him. Finally careful measurements are taken from the lower extremity of the anterior superior iliac spine to the upper margin of the patella

on either side. Quite possibly, especially if the manipulations have been leisurely and quiet, the length will already be nearly normal.

I notice that the first question usually asked is, "What prevents the occurrence of eversion?" The knee-sling prevents it. Upward lifting of the bent knee is the natural way of inverting the limb, when we wish to correct eversion; instinctively we first bend the knee and then lift it upwards. The practical fact is that eversion gives no trouble.

The usual weight required for an adult is 8 lb; for infants and older children $\frac{1}{2}$ lb to 4 lb. These weights, it will be noted, are doubled by the pulley arrangement nominally; but in practice it would seem that there is considerable modification of the pull one way and another, and considerable latitude within the range of efficiency. The truth seems to be that really a very moderate pull is adequate, provided that it is fairly constant and comfortable. At the end of the third week we always seek to reduce the weight.

The house surgeon's duty will be to take the measurements at least every morning and evening, and to inspect and adjust the pillows beneath the thigh and the leg so that there may be no backward sagging at the seat of fracture and the heel shall not be in contact with the bed. It is very little to require of him; but while it is very little and very easy, yet it is absolutely indispensable and must be faithfully given. The apparatus is far from being 'fool-proof' and cannot and will not look after itself.

One more word as to the significance of comfort. Comfort is the first essential in the treatment of a fracture. No apparatus that is not perfectly comfortable can be a good apparatus, for the muscles will never be at rest, but will always be striving to achieve a position of greater comfort. Moreover, there is, I am convinced, a direct relationship between comfort and rapid union, and an equally direct relationship between discomfort and delayed union, feeble union, and non-union. Explain this how we may, I have no doubt whatever about the clinical fact as a matter of bedside observation. Therefore let us never be content with any means, no matter how ingenious, and complicated, and satisfying to our theoretical preconceptions, that is not perfectly comfortable.

Esmarch's Bandage: Johann Friedrich August von Esmarch, 1823-1908

Esmarch was a military surgeon who was concerned with blood loss and first aid.

He was born at Tonning, Schleswig-Holstein, at a time when the province was struggling for freedom from Denmark. The son of a doctor, he studied at Gottingen and Kiel, becoming an assistant to Langenbeck.

It was during the insurrection against Denmark in 1848-50 that he began surgery—he also organised the resistance movement. In 1857 he became Professor of Surgery at Kiel, succeeding Stromeyer, the tenotomist, and marrying his daughter. He was engaged in military surgery again between 1866 and 1871 in the wars with Austria and France; in 1871 he became Surgeon General of the army. Soon after, in 1873, he married again—this time a Princess of Schleswig-Holstein. In the same year he published his description of the bandage that bears his name. He used this to produce a clear bloodless field for surgery and to diminish the blood loss during amputations in particular. His contributions to medicine were mainly derived from his battlefield experiences.

In 1869 and 1883 he published handbooks on First Aid and founded the Samaritan's Schools, based on the St. John's Ambulance Brigade, to teach First Aid throughout Germany.

"When I look back on my career as a surgeon I can say with truth that many and many are the times I have deplored that so very few people know how to render the first aid to those who have suddenly met with some injury. This specially applies to the field of battle; of the thousands who have flocked thither in their desire to help, so few have understood how to render aid."

His programme of education has improved the situation.

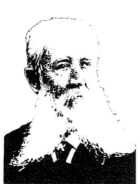

On the Artificial Emptying of Blood-Vessels in Operations: 1873

Gentlemen—You all witnessed yesterday a difficult and tedious operation, in which the patient lost a very large quantity of blood, in spite of all the care that was taken to prevent it.

What, more than all rendered the operation difficult, was the profuse haemorrhage. You will remember that, with almost every incision, although I took care to make them as slight as possible, one or more arteries spurted, or veins poured out their dark blood over the field of the operation. You saw how I sought to check the haemorrhage as much as possible by taking up the bleeding vessels, after each incision, with bulldog forceps, and left these hanging in the wound while I went on with the operation. More than once there were hanging in the wound all the twenty-four pairs of forceps which I always have at hand in great operations, and I was compelled first to tie the vessels already divided before I could cut deeper. When the operation was at last finished, I had applied altogether more than fifty ligatures, of which, however, fifteen were applied on the tumour itself, so that only thirty-five remained in the wound.

I cannot make any guess as to the exact quantity of blood lost, since it was constantly removed with sponges; but we could judge that the patient had very little blood left in her body by the wax-like paleness of the skin, the small, weak pulse, and the laboured respiration.

Most of you will, no doubt, have said to yourselves that you would not desire to commence your career as operators with such an extirpation. And, in fact, it is just the "demoniac" blood, as Dieffenbach called it, which not infrequently deters the young practitioner from performing an important operation, especially when he cannot command sufficient and reliable assistance. And yet he only becomes a good operator who has learnt calmly to enter into the struggle with haemorrhage. I need not explain to you here how important the question of haemorrhage is in almost every operation. In many cases the limit we put to our operative undertakings is determined by the extent of the haemorrhage to be expected. We do not venture to undertake many operations against which no other contra-indication exists, because the operation would last so long that we can foresee that the patient would bleed to death before it was completed, or because we consider him already too weak to survive the unavoidable loss of blood.

I shall perform an operation today in which the loss of blood would be still greater than in that of yesterday, if I did not adopt a procedure before commencing it which enables us to prevent the haemorrhage entirely. In the patient about to be placed upon the operating table, there is almost total necrosis of both tibiae, resulting from an acute osteo-myelitis, which followed a severe cold more than twenty years ago. You see that on the anterior surface of both legs numerous fistular openings exist, which discharge a large quantity of pus, and, through which the probe comes everywhere upon roughened, moveable bone. On handling the legs, you feel that the bones are enormously thickened, and from the long standing of the disease it may safely be assumed that the thickened bones, the case which contains the dead portion of bone (sequestrum), must also be of considerable hardness. The position of the fistulae, which you are extending on both legs almost from the upper to the lower epiphyses, justifies us in concluding that large portions of both diaphyses are dead, and the different depths at which sounds introduced into the fistulous openings come upon dead bone, indicate that the death of the bone at the different points occurred at different depths. If I leave a sound in each of these fistulous openings, and make a varying pressure with the upper sound upon the sequestrum, you see how all the other sounds are set in motion, and may fairly conclude therefrom that the entire sequestrum is moveable, and forms one continuous whole. To remove this, it is necessary to open the thickened bony case which contains it in its whole extent; and to ensure the complete healing of the large wound, I think it best to convert the bony cavity into a broad trough, by taking away the whole anterior wall, so that no adjacent cavities may remain to retard the healing process.

Those amongst you who have already seen similar operations will remember what profuse haemorrhage accompanied them, and how greatly the performance of them was rendered difficult and protracted by the loss of blood. Our patient is still tolerably well nourished, and not exactly to be called anaemic; but I do not believe that I should have ventured formerly to undertake both operations at one sitting, because I should have feared that the loss of blood would have placed the life of the patient in great danger. With the aid of the process which I am about to show you, I do not hesitate to undertake both the operations simultaneously, and to spare the patient thereby a second operation, and a second long confinement to bed. My assistant, Dr. Petersen, will operate upon the right leg at the same time and in the same manner as I do on the left. While the patient is being put under the influence of chloroform, the leg is first wrapped in waterproof varnished silk-paper, to prevent the bandages from being soiled by the discharge from the fistulous openings; both legs are then firmly bandaged from the points of the toes to above the knee with these elastic bandages, which are made of woven indiarubber, the uniform compression from which drives the blood out of the vessels of the limb. Immediately above the knee, where the bandage ends, we now apply this indiarubber tubing, well drawn out, four or five times round the thigh, and connect one end with the other by means of a hook and brass chain attached to them respectively. The indiarubber tubing so thoroughly compresses all the soft parts, including the arteries, that not a drop of blood can enter the part so treated. This has the special advantage over the tourniquet, that we can apply it at any part of the limb, and need not be concerned about the position of the main artery. Even in the most muscular and stoutest individuals we are able thoroughly to control the supply of blood by this simple process.

We now remove the bandages first applied, together with the varnished silk-paper, and you see that both legs below the tubing resemble completely those of a corpse and with their pale colour contrast almost uncomfortably with the rosy colour of the rest of the surface of the body. You will observe, also, that we operate precisely *as in the dead subject*.

We both now divide the soft parts along the whole anterior surface of the tibia down to the bone; a few drops of blood ooze from the bone and are wiped away with a sponge. From that time no more blood is seen. The periosteum, divided in the long direction, is now pushed back so far on both sides that the whole anterior surface of the thickened, uneven bone, with its numerous fistulous openings, is freely exposed.

We now take large chisels with wooden handles, such as are used by cabinet-makers, apply the edge to the uppermost fistulous opening, and, by the aid of a wooden hammer, remove the whole anterior surface of the bone in large chips.

The bone is very hard, as I expected. The work is not easy, and requires some practice, which you can best acquire in a joiner's shop. I must beg of you all to take care of your eyes, because the sharp and pointed splinters fly about with great force in all directions. We might remove this bony wall in another manner, with panel saws, or Heine's osteotome; but this is so much more laborious and tedious that I greatly prefer the chisel.

The large sequestrum now comes gradually more and more into sight. You can easily distinguish it, by its whitish colour, from the reddish, living bone. The difference of colour is, no doubt, much greater if you operate without cutting off the supply of blood to the parts; the blood then streams out of all the pores which you see on each newly-formed surface, as if from a sponge, sometimes in strong jets, and so completely fills the cavity of the wound at each blow of the chisel, that you recognise nothing more, and cannot use the chisel again until your assistant has thoroughly mopped out the cavity with sponges. But now I require no assistant; my assistant, Dr. Petersen, chisels out his cavity, like myself, in the sweat of his brow. And now the hardest work is done. Both sequestra are exposed to their whole extent; we seize them with powerful forceps and draw them out with some exertion, because they send a few irregular processes into lateral cavities.

You see that the large, trough-shaped cavities in the bones in which the sequestra lay are partly lined with pale-red granulations. We remove these with a sponge, which we press firmly upon and rub over the uneven, bony surface, and with small sharp scoops, with which we penetrate into the inlets and lateral cavities. We remove the granulations because they are, in my opinion, of no value for the reproduction of bone; they had been injured somewhat during the operation, so that they must have perished afterwards. You will be able to see, later on, that the whole surface of the bone very rapidly forms new luxuriant granulations, which soon become converted into bone-tissue and replace the great loss of substance.

The operation is now finished. We wash out the raw cavities with dilute carbolic acid, to destroy any decomposed organisms which may have got in, then put in some pieces of gauze steeped in a solution of chloride of iron, so as to cover the walls therewith, and now fill up both large cavities firmly with German tinder to above the level of the external skin. By bandaging with a strip of gauze dipped into carbolised oil, each of these pads is pressed well in; over this comes a layer of varnished silk-paper, air-tight round the whole leg, which is to be kept in its place with a common bandage.

We now, first, slowly remove the compressing indiarubber tubing. You see how the pale skin of the foot becomes red, first in spots, then uniformly everywhere, and soon even presents a darker red colour than the other parts of the body. Observe the dressing of the wound under the transparent paper; you nowhere see blood oozing through the gauze bandage. The patient has, therefore, not lost more than a teaspoonful of blood. And now, observe the still quietly sleeping patient; he has, even now, the same red cheeks as before the operation; his pulse is full and strong, and the recovery in his case will, no doubt, be much quicker and more certain than if we had removed the bone in the usual manner.

If we now compare the operation of today with that of yesterday, it will at once be evident to you how great are the advantages of this mode of proceeding, as well for the patient as for the operator. You have seen that we could both perform without assistance an operation difficult in itself, and will be convinced that this method will be very useful in ordinary practice, in which skilled assistance is often wanting.

You can adopt this method in almost all operations on the extremities with more or less complete success. In extirpations of tumours, tying of arteries, scraping out of scrofulous ulcers and carious bones, and in resections of smaller bones and joints, you can proceed in exactly the same manner as I have just shown you—i.e. you need not relax the compressing tubing until the dressing of the wound is completely finished.

I will now call your attention to another great advantage of this method. It consists therein that, in doubtful cases, where it is a question which is healthy, which diseased tissue, how far our active interference must extend, whether we must amputate or endeavour to proceed conservatively, resect, scrape off, etc., we are enabled by this method to examine the diseased parts much more minutely than would otherwise be possible. In many cases in which I was obliged to propose to the patients an amputation of the leg above the ankle, on account of disease in the ankle-joint, I have promised them, before administering chloroform, first to examine the diseased parts very minutely, and to save the foot if I thought it possible to do so. After driving out the blood as above, I have treated the foot exactly as on the dissecting-room table; have laid free and examined minutely the diseased bones and joints and only performed the amputation when I had convinced myself that it was impossible to preserve the part, without the patient's having lost a drop of blood until I had tied all the arteries visible to the naked eye. Then only have I removed the tubing and tied the smaller arteries from which blood came.

I must observe generally, that amputations and larger resections of the joints cannot be carried out so completely without loss of blood, as in the operation you have just witnessed, because we must ensure ourselves against after-haemorrhage before we dress the wound. If you amputate, you must relax the tubing as soon as you have taken up all the arteries which you can recognise as such with the naked eye. The blood now rushes at first with great force into the vessels and flows for a moment, as if out of a sponge, over the whole surface of the wound. Very soon, however, you distinguish single spirting arteries, and when you have taken up these you are pretty safe from after-haemorrhage, because, from the dilatation of vessels caused by the removal of the tubing, even the smallest arteries show themselves at once, and no branch of any size can easily be overlooked.

In no case is the loss of blood great, and the results of amputation here have been extremely favourable since I employed the method described above.

As in the extremities, so you can entirely cut off the supply of blood to the male genital organs by means of indiarubber tubing. If you wish to remove a testicle or to amputate the penis, you apply a thin indiarubber tubing from behind round the root of the scrotum and penis, cross the ends in front of the mons veneris, and tie them on the loins. In this way I have often performed castration, as well as amputation of the penis, without losing more than the modicum of blood which is to be found in those organs before the commencement of the operation. If you would avoid even this, you must first apply narrow elastic bandages carefully to the parts, which would be very desirable in the case of large tumours of the scrotum. For slighter operations upon the prepuce or glans, it suffices to place once round the root of the penis a piece of very thin indiarubber tubing, such as is used for draining wounds and abscesses.

With the so manifold and successful employment of indiarubber in surgery, it lay near at hand to use its elasticity for our present purpose, and it proved efficient beyond all expectation. As soon as it was ascertained that we could very easily completely interrupt the circulation with an ordinary indiarubber tubing the present method developed itself very quickly.

Tubing, such as is used for counter-extension in the weight-treatment of inflamed joints, served at first as a tourniquet, and one of those indiarubber bandages with which we are enabled so rapidly to disperse dropsical effusions into the knee-joint, was used for bandaging the extremity. With every trial I made of the new method its advantages became more apparent. One improvement was tried after the other. The more I became convinced of the great advantages of the method, the more desirous I was to extend it to as many operations as possible. The field is, unfortunately, a very narrow one. We can prevent, the access of blood completely in the extremities only, and external organs of generation in the male.

But the tubing may perhaps be found useful in operations on the trunk, neck, and head, by shutting off the blood of all, or some of the extremities from the general circulation, by strapping, and thus forming reserve stores from which we could admit the blood successively again into the general circulation if the patient was in danger of bleeding to death. This is, however, an idea only, the practicability of which careful experiments on men and animals can alone determine.

I cherish the hope, however, that this method may yet be available in many directions, but must, in conclusion, ask one question which is of the greatest importance with regard to its introduction, namely, whether dangers may not arise to the health of the patient from the employment of it. In any case, we must not ignore the possibility that the firm strapping of a limb for any considerable length of time may be followed by dangerous derangements of the circulation and innervation, such as thromboses, inflammations, paralyses, etc.

After the thousandfold experiences, however, which the surgeons of all times and of all countries have had in the employment of the tourniquet and of compression with the fingers, it was not exactly probable that an interruption of the circulation, even if complete, could be followed by such evil consequences, unless continued for a great length of time. And if the carefully performed experiments of Cohnheim have shown that in warm-blooded animals, the total interruption of the circulation of the blood is not in general followed by any permanent disturbance, if it does not continue more than six or eight hours, I may now, after having performed during the last year more than eighty operations on parts artificially emptied of their blood, assure you that I also have never seen such disturbances ensue which could be pointed out as consequences of the method in question. I have performed operations which lasted more than an hour, and have not found that, during the recovery, any disturbances of the circulation showed themselves; on the other hand, it is seen that the wounds made during the operation ran a strikingly favourable course since I have adopted this method, and accidental, traumatic affections occur only exceptionally. There is one precaution which I would urge you strongly to take when adopting this method. If you are operating upon parts infiltrated with ichorous matter, you must refrain from emptying them completely of their blood. If you bandaged such soft parts tightly, you would be in danger of driving the infectious matters into the meshes of the cellular tissue and extremities of the lymphatic vessels, and might possibly do much harm thereby.

In such cases I do not put on the bandage at all, but content myself, before applying the tubing, with emptying the limbs as completely as possible of blood, by causing it to be raised high in the air for a few moments.

2 OPERATIONS ON BONE

Corrective Osteotomy: John Rhea Barton, 1794-1871

It is unusual for a surgeon to develop two entirely new principles of treatment and to realise the significance of the innovations himself. Barton introduced both arthroplasty and corrective osteotomy for limb deformities. His ideas have been elaborated and applied to a wide range of situations.

He was born in Lancaster, Pennsylvania, the son of a Judge, and studied at the Pennsylvania Hospital. He later worked for the Father of American Surgery, Dr. Physick, who was one of Hunter's pupils, before being elected to the surgical staff himself at the age of 29.

He is said to have possessed great manual dexterity, and was ambidextrous, with the result that once he had positioned himself for an operation he was not always shunting about.

In 1854 he wired a fractured patella, but lost the patient from sepsis. His name is occasionally attached to a fracture he described—carpal sub-luxation with a marginal fracture of the articular surface of the radius.

A New Treatment for Ankylosis: Barton, 1837

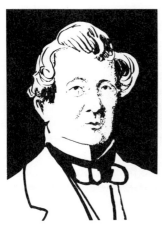

The object of my treatment was to remove deformity, and to restore to usefulness a limb which had unfortunately been suffered to become anchylosed in a mal-position. The following will, I trust, satisfactorily explain the operation and the after treatment of the case, as well as the principles by which I was guided in the management of it.

S—— D——'s, M.D., formerly of Charleston, S.C., but now a resident of Alabama, when a youth of about nine years of age unluckily had his knee joint involved in inflammation and suppuration so extensively as to occasion the destruction of the synovial membranes, the ligaments, cartilages, and in short, every structure peculiarly appertaining to the joint. After a protracted suffering he finally recovered with the loss of the joint; the tibia, femur and patella having become united to each other in the form of a true anchylosis. The loss of the articulation of the knee, however, though a misfortune, did not constitute the *sadness* of his case. It was caused by the mal-position of the limb; the leg having been flexed upon the thigh to a degree somewhat less than a right angle. Hence the only alternatives of which he could avail himself to aid him in walking were, either to use crutches, or to employ a very high block-sole boot, and to lower his stature by flexing the sound limb, in order that both feet might reach the ground. The latter expedient he adopted. The long continued pressure and weight of the body sustained by this defective limb, acting under such great mechanical disadvantages, had at length caused some projection of the instep, and other irregularities, which it is unnecessary to particularise.

This supposed irremediable condition of his limb, with all its ills, the young gentleman endured during the period of about sixteen years. In the meantime he graduated in medicine, and became a successful and highly respectable practitioner; but as his professional labours increased, he found the condition of his limb to be an obstacle not only to his further success, but also a source of unceasing annoyance and vexation. Whereupon, with a resoluteness not surprising to those who knew the strength of his mind, the firmness of his character, and the abundance of his manly courage, he repaired to Philadelphia in order that some relief might be obtained, if it were possible. When consulted by him I found him fully prepared to learn that no benefit was to be expected from any heretofore known practice, and that if he could be relieved it must be by some novel expedient and treatment.

After a candid and full disclosure of my views of his case, and of the means by which I thought he might be benefited, his own judgment accorded with mine; and believing in the feasibility of the plans, he became urgent for the undertaking. It was accordingly commenced on the 27th day of May, 1835, and pursued as follows:-

Two incisions were made over the femur, just above the patella. The first commenced at a point opposite the upper and anterior margin of the external condyle of the femur, and, passing obliquely across the front of the thigh, terminated on the inner side. The second incision commenced also on the outer side, about two and a half inches above the first; and passing likewise obliquely across the thigh, terminated with the other in an acute angle. By these incisions were divided the integuments, the tendon of the extensor muscles of the leg, at its insertion into the upper part of the patella, and some of the contiguous fibres of the rectus and crureus muscles themselves, a greater part of the vastus internus, and a portion of the vastus externus muscles. A flap, composed therefore of this structure, was elevated from the femur close to the condyles. The soft parts were next detached from the outer side of the bone, from the base of the flap toward the ham, by passing a knife over the circumference of it, so as to admit of the use of a saw. The flap then being turned aside a triangular or wedge-like piece of the femur was easily removed by means of a small narrow bladed saw; such as was used in the operation at the hip. This wedge of bone did not include the entire diameter of the femur at the point of section; so that a few lines of the posterior portion of the shaft of the bone remained yet undivided. By slightly inclining the leg backward, these yielded, and the solution was complete. This mode of effecting the lesion of the bone was designedly adopted, and constituted what I conceived to be a very important measure in the operation. Important, because it rendered a popliteal artery free from the danger of being wounded by the action of the saw, and subsequently the interlocking of the fractured surfaces tended to retain the extremities of the divided bone in their positions until the harshness of their surfaces had been overcome either by the absorption of their angles, or by the deposition of new matter upon them—a change essential to the safety of the artery during the subsequent treatment of the case. Not a blood-vessel was opened which required either a ligature or compression. The operation, which lasted about five minutes, being thus ended, the

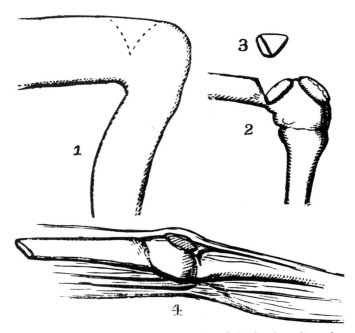

Barton: Osteotomy. 1. Gives the position of the flap just above the knee; 2. Shows the operation on the femur; 3. The piece of bone removed; 4. The manner in which the gap in the bone was closed by the overlapping of the surfaces consequent to the extension of the leg. These uniting restored the integrity of the limb.

reflected flap was restored to its place, the wound lightly dressed, and the patient was put to bed. lying on his back, with the limb supported upon a splint of *an angle corresponding to that of the knee previous to the operation.* This position was maintained until it was believed that the asperities of the bone had become blunted, and were not likely by their pressure to cause ulceration of the artery beneath them. This first splint was then removed, and another having the angle slightly obtuse was substituted. In a few days a third splint, with the angle more obtuse than that of the second, supplied its place. Others, varying in degrees of angularity, in like manner came in their turn to support the limb until it had attained a position almost straight. It was then unchangeably continued in that line until the contact surfaces of the bone had united and securely fixed the limb in this the desired direction.

During the treatment of the case, especial care was bestowed in protecting the popliteal vessels against any injurious encroachment upon them. With that view, all antagonising pressure on the soft parts in the ham was carefully avoided. The limb was rested on two longbran bags, laid upon the splint, with their ends apart—a vacancy of four or five inches being left between them opposite the lesion of the bone. This interspace was lightly filled with carded cotton, so as to afford a safe support. Every symptom of pain or uneasiness in this part was promptly attended to. The occasional issue of a drop or two of blood from the corner of the sore, during the process of dressing the limb, caused me some solicitude in this case; whereas, ordinarily I should have considered it as a matter of no moment—it being so frequent an occurrence during the dressing of wounds, owing to the disturbance of the granulations, especially in compound fractures. The wounded soft parts finally healed and quieted his anxiety. The straightening of the limb having been very cautiously and by degrees effected, the first two months elapsed during the accomplishment of this object. Having then reduced it to the desired position, means were carefully observed to retain it so until the reunion of the bone had been fully completed; which occupied two months longer. The constitutional symptoms were such as usually occur in compound fractures—somewhat severe, but at no time alarming. Throughout the whole treatment it was not found necessary to bleed him, or to have recourse to any very active constitutional measures. He was occasionally indisposed from irregularity in the digestive functions, but was always speedily relieved by resorting to mild and appropriate remedies.

At the end of about four months from the date of the operation my patient stood erect, with both feet in their natural position, and the heels resting alike upon the floor, although a slight angle had been designedly left at the knee, in order that there might not be any necessity for throwing the limb out from the body in the act of walking, which is always the case when the knee is quite straight. After this period, the use of shoes of the ordinary shape was resumed, and the limb was daily exercised with increasing strength and usefulness. On the 19th of October, the Doctor took his departure for the South, bearing with him the injunction to continue the support of a small splint and the aid of a crutch or cane, until he should acquire sufficient confidence in the strength of the limb to justify him in laying them aside.

I was subsequently advised of his improvement; but was resolved not to give publicity to the case until the full and entire benefit of the operation could be ascertained. The wide distance which afterwards separated us prevented me from obtaining the necessary and direct information until within a recent period. I have the pleasure now not only to afford this intelligence, but to present it in the most satisfactory manner. Having written to the doctor for the information, and to learn from him in what manner it might be agreeable that I should refer to him as the subject of the case, the following clear, satisfactory, and well-written answer was promptly received. As the letter is full of interest in the case, I must be excused if I publish it almost entire, even though it contain some flattering sentiments for the one to whom it is addressed. That part only has been omitted which is in courtesy to my family.

Charleston, November 6th, 1837.

"My dear sir,

. . . I have the satisfaction and pleasure of saying to you now, that the operation you performed on my leg has been *completely* successful, and has more than realised my most sanguine anticipations. The small abscess, which you dressed the day before we parted at Norfolk, continued open, and threw out, from time to time, small pieces of bone, until the August after, when the last piece was discharged; the orifice then closed, and I have suffered no material inconvenience from it since. From the January previous, however, I was going about and attending to my professional business; and early in the summer, when our sickly season commenced, I was on horseback daily, riding from thirty to fifty miles a day; without more than the ordinary fatigue or inconvenience. I am at present well; the wound sound; and I feel no other inconvenience in riding or walking, than what arises from my knee joint being stiff, which was the case before you performed the operation. I walk without a stick or other aid, with the sole of the foot to the ground, and my friends tell me, with but a slight limp; and I have great pleasure in adding that the leg and foot have increased considerably in size, so as now to be nearly equal to the other. When I think of what I was, and what I am; and that to your firmness, judgment, and skill, I am indebted for the happy change, I want words to express adequately all that I feel. I will not attempt it, but believe me, my dear sir, I feel it not the less.

I shall remain here for a week or two longer, and if you wish any further information on my case, do write me, and I will give it most cheerfully. After that period I cannot say where a letter would reach me. Adieu . . . .
. . . .
and am, my dear sir, very sincerely, your friend,

Seaman Deas.

To Dr. J. Rhea Barton.

In 1845 Gurdon Buck improved on this procedure. Barton's operation produced angular deformity just above the knee so that the line of the tibia was some inches in front of the femur. The artist who drew Barton's illustration has concealed this by extending the leg at the knee joint and not at the osteotomy.

Buck performed the osteotomy through the knee joint.

Corrective Osteotomy: Mayer, 1853

OPERATION FOR KNOCK-KNEES

To the Editor of *The Lancet*

Sir,

The following case of operation for *knock-knees* is reported by Dr. Mayer, of the Orthopaedic Hospital at Wurzburg, in the proceedings of the Medical Society of that place (lately published), and seems well worth recording in your pages.

Your most obedient servant,

Knightsbridge, April, 1853.   F. A. B. Bonney.

John II——, a strong and healthy-looking boy of fifteen, son of a baker, and employed in his father's business, was found, on admission into the Orthopaedic Hospital at Wurzburg, to have the right leg diverging about seven inches, and the left about eight, from the direction of the corresponding thigh, as seen in the first figure of the accompanying sketch.

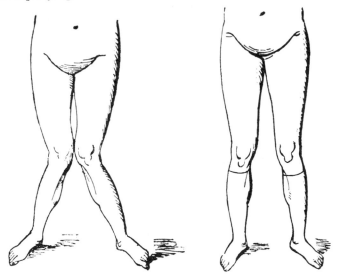

Mayer: Osteotomy

On the 14th of August, 1851, the lad having been put under the influence of chloroform. Dr. Mayer made an incision beginning three-quarters of an inch below the insertion of the ligamentum patellae, and curving downwards so as nearly to surround the front and inner (or mesial) side of the head of the tibia. He then turned the flap upwards, and divided the periosteum in the line of the first incision, and afterwards, with Heine's cutting-needle, separated the periosteum from the outer and posterior surface of the tibia, so as to prepare for the use of the saw. To protect the soft parts in that situation during the sawing, a strip of watch-spring, about half an inch wide was introduced between the denuded bone and the periosteum. Dr. Mayer, then, with a round saw, made two incisions converging towards the posterior part of the tibia, and meeting about a line and a half from the surface, without therefore quite cutting the bone in two. The wedge thus excised was about five lines thick at its base, and was easily removed by forceps. The wound was cleared of bone-dust by forcible injections of cold water, after which, through the flexibility of the remaining isthmus of the tibia and the mobility of the fibula, no difficulty was found in bringing the cut surfaces of bone into close apposition. The outer wound was brought together with the greatest accuracy by needles and ligatures (as for hare-lip), the haemorrhage being quite inconsiderable. The leg was then put into one of Boyer's hollow splints, used for fracture of the patella.

Half an hour after the operation as, through the perfect apposition of the divided parts, no discharge of any kind was visible, the wound was covered with a thick layer of collodium, and upon this drying the ligature and needles were removed. The traumatic reaction was very slight, and on the fourth day the external wound (five inches long) had perfectly united. The leg was now left quiet in the splint for twenty-three days, when Dr. Mayer had the pleasure of finding that the incised surfaces of bone had united also. The next day the patient was allowed to walk in his room with crutches, and a few days afterwards in the garden without any artificial support whatever.

On the 3rd of October the other leg was operated on in the same manner and with the same success. He left the hospital, free from deformity, and with a firm and natural gait, on the 19th of November.

Macewen's Osteotomy: Sir William Macewen, 1848–1924

The youngest of 12 children, William Macewen was born on the Isle of Bute and graduated from Glasgow in the time of Lister and Syme. At the age of 28 he was elected to the surgical staff of the Royal Infirmary.

The new concept of antiseptic surgery was quickly assimilated by Macewen and enabled him to work up experimental operations so that they were safe, gave consistent results, and were no longer a desperate remedy but a widely applicable technique. For example, in 1877 he first performed subcutaneous osteotomy for genu valgum using an antiseptic technique; only seven years later he reported a series of 1800 osteotomies for this condition without any serious infection in a single case. There were, of course, a large number of cases of rickets in Glasgow at this time.

He found a chisel unsuitable for cutting bone transversely and devised a special instrument sharpened on both surfaces so that it did not deviate to one side, for which he coined the word "osteotome".

He was a pioneer of chest surgery and neurosurgery and introduced bone grafting. Bone growth was his main research interest and he made many contributions; he made a special study of antler formation to further his knowledge of prodigious rates of bone growth.

Macewen's Osteotomy: 1878

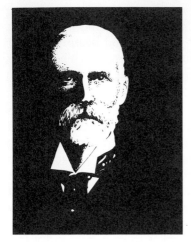

Clinical Lecture on

ANTISEPTIC OSTEOTOMY

Delivered at the Royal Infirmary, Glasgow by

William Macewen, M.D.

Surgeon and Lecturer on Clinical Surgery at the Infirmary

Gentlemen,

For some time past those of you who attend my wards have seen under treatment two patients on whom osteotomy was performed for the relief of knock-knee; and, as I intend performing a similar operation this morning, you will allow me to bring the subject of antiseptic osteotomy briefly under your notice.

We may date the introduction of osteotomy, in its modern acceptation from the time when a firm faith in the value of anti-septics had gained possession of the minds of some surgeons who saw that they thus possessed a power enabling them with safety and surety to undertake operations which otherwise would be so dangerous to life that they were never contemplated. The credit of first performing antiseptic osteotomy in its scientific spirit is due to Professor Volkmann, of Holle. Within a few days after receiving Volkmann's brochure containing two cases of antiseptic osteotomy, an instance of anchylosis of the knee came under my notice, closely resembling those spoken of by that celebrated German surgeon; and as this turned out to be my first case of osteotomy, you will permit me to refer to it in a few words.

In the month of March, 1875, I was consulted by the parents of a girl, six years of age, who was affected with a stiff bent leg. Her father stated that she had had scarlet fever about a year previously, and that as a sequela her right knee-joint suppurated, causing her great pain, which became excruciating whenever the limb was attempted to be stretched. Not foreseeing the consequence, she was allowed to keep the limb flexed until the pain had subsided, when it was discovered that the knee-joint was stiff, and the limb could not be stretched, thus rendering her unfit to walk except by the aid of a crutch. She had a delicate appearance. The right lower limb was flexed at the knee to nearly a right angle and anchylosed, though permitting a perceptible amount of motion. The patella was fixed to the outer, and partly to the under, surface of the femur. The affected limb was smaller than its neighbour, and the measurement showed fully half an inch of shortening. Forcible straightening was here out of the question. I therefore determined to perform an osteotomy. On April 11th, 1875, I removed a wedge-shaped portion of bone from the anterior surface of the femur; the posterior layers were then fractured, and the leg straightened though, as the joint was stiff, it was considered expedient to keep the limb slightly flexed, as in that position it would be more convenient for sitting, and at the same time would interfere little with her walking. The wound was dressed and the limb put up in plaster-of-Paris, windows being left for dressing. The parts healed as a typically aseptic wound does. There was no redness about the wound, no pus, no fever, no constitutional disturbance. In May she was removed from her lodging in Glasgow to her own home in the country, where, toward the middle of June, she was able to walk about, the bone being then firmly united. Now she walks easily, without a stick or other support, though with a slight limp.

This, then, gentlemen, as far as I am aware, was the first.

Case 2. A. R., aged eighteen years, came under observation in May 1877, suffering from an aggravated state of genu-valgum. He was a pale, delicate-looking lad, with soft tissues and feeble pulse. His parents and family were healthy, though he represented one of his sisters as having weak ankles. He first became affected when he was nine years of age, and the knees have gradually inclined more and more till within the last six months, when he was reduced to such a state that he could neither walk nor stand for more than five minutes at once, and even during that time he suffered considerable pain. He was unable to stand on one leg. When asked to stand, he crossed one limb in front of the other, the one foot resting on the outer side of the dorsum of the other foot. Both when standing and walking he kept his body bent well forward. He could not walk without a stick or support. His walk was laboured and evidently distressing, the one knee having to circumnavigate the other in a cumbrous fashion. His feet were inverted as they met the ground, and his toes grasped the surface of the floor, in an attempt to steady himself. The internal condyles measured fully an inch in length more than the external condyles. The patellae were thrown outwards, and the patellar articular surfaces of the femora were exposed. The heads of the tibiae were also enlarged.

Under these circumstances he was desirous that something should be done for his relief. Owing to his weak constitutional state, I would have preferred sending him to the country for a time before operating, but as he was unfit to take anything like exercise, I determined to operate on one limb at once. This was done on May 19th. An incision was made over the inner condyle of the right femur, the centre of which corresponded with the upper part of the condyle, my object being to go as near to the joint as possible without opening into it. A V-shaped portion of bone was struck out by the chisel from the inner side of the condyloid extremity of the femur, the remainder of the bone was broken, and the limb was brought round straight. The operation and after-treatment were conducted antiseptically. During the first fortnight there was an oozing of blood and serum, afterwards there was a distinct discharge of pus, though very small and perfectly sweet. The limb was placed in a half box-splint, the foot being elevated. As this was the first case of osteotomy for *knock-knee* which I had performed, I kept him in the hospital for a longer time than I now see was necessary. He was dismissed with a firm strong limb and a perfectly mobile knee-joint. As he was then able to walk, he went to the country to recruit, and did not return until November to have the other limb operated on. He was then improved in health and much pleased with his one straight leg.

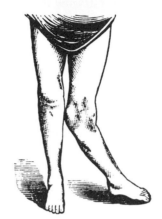 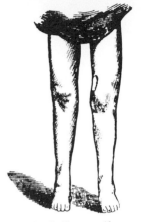

After first operation on right leg; the left leg in natural state.　　　After both operations.

These woodcuts are taken from photographs.

Macewen: Osteotomy

On the 17th November, 1877, the left limb was operated on in the same manner as above described. It was afterwards put up in a paraffin splint, with a small window cut in it for reapplication of the dressings. This splint acted well, and was very easy and comfortable. This time also there was a purulent discharge, though slight and aseptic. At the end of the fourth week, the paraffin splint was removed, and the bone was found firm. A support of Gooch was then applied to the outside of the limb. It was removed at the end of the sixth week, when he was allowed to get out of bed.

You will observe that in this case suppuration took place after both operations. I attribute this, partly at least, to the wounds having been closed with sutures immediately after the operation, although there was a drainage-tube also inserted. In my first osteotomy the wound was left open, and it healed by vitalisation of the blood clot between its lips; and in the case which I will show you next the same thing happened after similar treatment of the wound. But although in this lad's case there was slight suppuration, there was at no time any inflammatory blush round the part, and no constitutional disturbance. His rectal temperature on the second day after the operation being 100.6°, and it gradually decreased from that date. Now, as you see him, his legs are straight, he can flex his knee-joints, he walks without a support, and he feels very happy at the result. (See Fig. 2.) When his clothes are on, no one would surmise that he had once been the subject of knock-knee. In this instance the operations were not performed as a mere convenience, but as an absolute necessity in order to allow of locomotion, as you remember he could neither stand nor walk for more than five consecutive minutes prior to the operation.

He describes two further cases which healed primarily.

Bone Grafting

For nearly three centuries osseous defects have been replaced by bone grafts. Perhaps the first person to do this was Jobi Meekren in 1682. He replaced a defect in the cranium of a soldier with a piece of dog's skull; the implant is said to have healed in perfectly. However Jobi Meekren was required by the church authorities to remove the graft, under the ban of excommunication, as they refused to recognise such unchristian methods of treatment. This is recorded, not in the surgical literature, but in church records.

At the beginning of the nineteenth century several surgeons transplanted bone with occasional success. A little later in the century Ollier performed a great volume of experimental work but was discouraged because his grafts were absorbed through being put in the soft tissues. Bone grafting, though it was clearly possible, did not become a practicality until the advent of antiseptic surgery. Macewen, who had studied under Lister and was fascinated by bone growth, produced some spectacular results and a few surgeons copied him with varying success.

It was in about 1911 that bone grafting became an accepted technique due to the work of Fred Albee of New York (1876-1945). Albee used cortical bone grafts accurately carpentered to produce a cabinet-maker's joint. He moved away from the tools of a sculptor and introduced electrical saws. Looking back it is surprising that bone grafting should have come into its own with cortical grafts as these are looked upon today as not only more difficult to insert but also less reliable than cancellous grafting.

Phemister in 1931 wrote the paper that coupled his name with cancellous grafting of ununited fractures. But in fact the paper is a very matter of fact comparison of different methods of treatment rather than an encouraging account. In 1933 Ghormley used iliac grafts for lumbo-sacral fusion but few surgeons followed him. The value of cancellous bone grafting was not widely appreciated until the Second World War when, perhaps, fixation was better and the graft was not required to provide both fixation and new bone. Rainsford Mowlem, a plastic surgeon, showed the clear supremacy of cancellous grafting for ununited fractures for the first time in 1944.

It seems likely that alternatives to bone grafting as a means of stimulating the growth will be found in the future. If, as Macewen pointed out, deer can produce new bone to form a new pair of antlers in a few months, then some easier method than grafting should be possible.

OBSERVATIONS CONCERNING TRANSPLANTATION OF BONE
Illustrated by a case of inter-human osseous transplantation whereby over two thirds of the shaft of the humerus was restored:

William Macewen: 1881

William Connell, aged three years, was admitted into the Royal Infirmary, Glasgow, under my care, on the 17 July 1878, in a much emaciated and exhausted condition arising from suppuration in connection with necrosis of the right humerus. On August 7, 1878, the part of the necrosed bone exposed at the operation was divided by the bone forceps. The upper part of the shaft was then caught by lion forceps, rotated in order to loosen its periosteal attachments, and then pulled out. The lower portion was similarly dealt with.

The arm healed but was useless and the parents wanted amputation, but Macewen encouraged them to allow him to try to improve it.

Transplantation of two wedges of bone on November 9, 1879 (one year and three months after the removal of the necrosed shaft); an incision was made down to the extremity of the upper fragment. This extremity was found to be cartilaginous for fully a quarter of an inch. This cartilaginous spike was removed leaving then a portion of bone which measured $1\frac{3}{4}$ inches from the tip of the acromion process. From this point a sulcus about 2 inches in length was made in a downward direction between the muscles. The former presence of bone was nowhere indicated and the sole guide as to the correct position into which the transplant was to be placed was an anatomical one. After the sulcus was formed, the haemorrhage was fully arrested and an aseptic sponge was placed in the gap, which was then ready to receive the bone.

Two wedges were then removed from the tibia of a patient six years of age, affected with anterior tibial curves. The last of these osseous wedges consisted of the anterior portion of the tibia, along with its periosteum, the wedges gradually tapering towards the posterior part of the tibia.

They were removed, then cut into small fragments with the chisel, and immediately thereafter deposited into the sulcus in the boy's arm. They were kept under the spray while they were removed from the tibia until they were covered by the soft parts of the arm and its antiseptic dressing. . . . (He repeated the graft on Feb. 1 and July 9, 1880).

At the beginning of March 1881 the bone was found firmly united, from the head to the condyles, and measured 6 inches, while the left humerus measured $6\frac{1}{2}$ inches, that is to say $\frac{1}{2}$ an inch longer than the transplanted one. The patient could lift his arm to his head and otherwise use it.

Macewen published a follow up note in 1909.

It is now thirty years since the humeral shaft was rebuilt and during the greater part of this period the man has depended on his physical exertions for the earning of his livelihood. He has worked as a joiner for many years and is now an engineer's pattern maker. His grafted arm has increased in length but not proportionate to the sound one. Measurements: The grafted humerus measures from the tip of the acromium to the tip of the external condyle 10″ but following the curve in the bone it is 11″ long. The sound humerus from the same points measures 14″- 3″ longer than the other.

After this William Connell served in the First World War.

Internal Fixation: Sir William Arbuthnot Lane, 1856-1938

Arbuthnot Lane was a superb technician, and this was to some extent his downfall—operating became safe and enabled him to perform hundreds of colectomies for constipation.

He was born at Inverness, the son of an army surgeon, and began to study at Guy's Hospital at the age of 16. For the first six years after qualifying, apart from a period as a ship's surgeon, he studied in the dissecting room, trying to relate occupation to skeletal form. Conan Doyle is said to have had him in mind to some extent when he created Sherlock Holmes. He paid great attention to the effects of fractures on joint form. The deleterious effect of mal-union on the joint and the earning capacity of the patient led him to undertake internal fixation of fractures. In 1892 he originated the "no touch" technique, which is used today, to make surgery safe. After screwing a few fractures of the tibia with success, he proceeded to screw all those he came across in order to show other surgeons that it could be done and that it was safe. The metal he used was ordinary steel, which became corroded—fortunately the film of rust which formed acted to some extent as an insulator, preventing gross oxidation. If dissimilar metals are used this does not form, and a severe electrolyte reaction occurs, leading to destruction of the metal and inflammation of the tissues. In 1905 he started to use plates. Though internal fixation had been used sporadically for almost a century before in the form of bronze and silver wire, it was Arbuthnot Lane who made internal fixation a practical procedure, and wrote a book about his methods.

He was always a general surgeon, and was one of the first to open the mastoid antrum for an infected mastoid, and resect part of a rib for empyema. The enthusiasm he brought to colonic surgery was his chief claim to fame. It was his opinion that diseases such as tuberculosis of bone, rheumatoid arthritis, and many other conditions were largely due to constipation, and he treated them by ileo-colostomy. He removed colons wholesale; he introduced liquid paraffin to the pharmocopoea. Finally he realised he could not cope with the therapeutic problem he had set himself and started a programme of health education. He started columns in the papers, public lectures, and the New Health Society. Those who today think the public well educated about medicine can congratulate or blame the originator as they wish. Lane resigned from the Medical Register before embarking on this so that he could not be accused of unethical conduct. He raised money to found the first Chair of Dietetics, and improved the distribution of fruit and vegetables.

Though the things he was most devoted to seem to have been the triumph of technique over reason, he started a new era of fracture treatment.

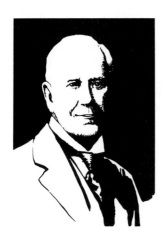

A method of treating Simple Oblique Fractures of the Tibia and Fibula more efficient than those in common use

by W. Arbuthnot Lane, M.S., 1894

My experience of the usual methods of treating simple oblique fractures of the tibia and fibula in certain classes of labouring men, by manipulation of the fragments and the subsequent retention of the limb in some form of splint, is that the results so obtained are but too frequently unsatisfactory in the extreme.

I do not allude to the presence of any considerable shortening or deformity, for with moderate skill and care such conditions can be generally avoided, though in some cases deformity and shortening are noticeable features. In this paper I will confine myself solely to the consideration of the physical capacity of the man to perform his accustomed heavy work after he has sustained an oblique fracture of both bones of the leg, or in other words of his relative financial value as a machine, both before and after the accident, and I have no hesitation whatever in asserting that, under the methods of treatment at present adopted, not only is the man totally incapacitated from earning a living for an unnecessarily long period, but in a considerable proportion of cases he is unable subsequently to perform such heavy work as he was able to do before the injury, so that he is obliged to follow some less remunerative pursuit, if indeed he has not to depend solely on charity. In fact, his machinery is financially depreciated by the accident, occasionally to the extent of at least 70 to 80 per cent. of its original value.

If what I state is true, the form of treatment of such fractures which is universally adopted in our hospitals is simply disastrous, and can only be perpetuated because we are unaware of the financial loss or even ruin which our very imperfect surgical methods entail on our unfortunate patients. Though the shortening and deformity are usually trifling, the somewhat complicated displacement of the ends of the fragments on one another is sufficient to completely alter, and often irretrievably damage, the machinery of the lower extremity. The deviation of the axes of the lower fragments of the tibia and fibula from the directions they originally occupied when in continuity with the upper portions of the respective bones causes pressure to be transmitted through the joints of the ankle and foot, of the knee, and to some extent even of the hip, in such an abnormal manner that the individual experiences not only a feeling of insecurity in these joints, which is especially marked in the foot and ankle, but he also suffers from progressively increasing pain and discomfort.

This means that the anatomy of the several joints which are called upon to perform a function other than that they were accustomed to carry out must alter in consequence of, and in proportion to, the degree in which the directions of the lines of pressure which is transmitted through the joints are changed.

Under these altered circumstances the joints are unable to carry out their physiological functions with the same accuracy and perfection that they did previous to the accident, and this inability is a progressive one, and is accompanied by pain and discomfort which increases rapidly, and is most marked in those who sustain such fractures when past middle age.

There are many other troubles which the patient experiences because of his inability to use the muscles and joints of his leg with the same accuracy, ease, and freedom as before, such as oedema, eczema, ulceration, etc.

Even if there is only a small proportion of truth in what I assert —and in my opinion my experience justifies me in making the assertion—it is obvious folly to continue our present methods of treatment, especially as more effectual means are ready to hand.

Why should we hesitate for one moment to bring common sense mechanical principles to bear in the case of simple fractures of the tibia and fibula, when most surgeons of the present day would not dream of doing otherwise in the case of fracture of the patella with separation of fragments? May I ask this question: are we able by operative measures to treat oblique fractures of the tibia and fibula so that there shall be no alteration from the normal in the lines of pressure through the several joints? in other words, can we restore the bones to their original form? This can certainly be done, and at a minimum risk to the patient, by freely exposing the fragments at the seat of fracture, by bringing the surfaces into accurate apposition, and retaining them permanently in that position.

Such operative measures offer to the patient the following advantages:

(a) They at once relieve him from the pain of any movement of the fragments upon one another.

(b) They free him from the tension and discomfort due to the extensive extravasation of blood between and into the tissues.

(c) They shorten the duration of the period during which he is incapacitated from work, since union is practically by first intention, and consequently very rapid and perfect.

(d) Lastly, and by far the most important, they leave his skeletal mechanics in the condition in which they were before he sustained the injury.

The two questions which now arise are:

"Is much difficulty experienced in bringing the surfaces into accurate apposition?" and "What is the best method of retaining them in that apposition?"

In answer to the first question, it is often very difficult, even when the tibial fracture is freely exposed, to bring the surfaces into apposition by means of manipulation of the limb and of the broken ends, but in every case in which I have used screw pressure I have succeeded in doing so. At the same time it is obvious that even though by these means the surgeon may fail in obtaining perfectly accurate apposition, he will get union with very much less displacement than with the ordinary methods, and consequently, a correspondingly better result.

Now as regards the best means of fixation of the fragments: in my earlier cases I used silver wire, but soon gave it up, as it was open to two great objections. Firstly, as it is necessary to fasten its ends, it could only be passed in certain directions with safety, and to secure it satisfactorily one was at times obliged to incise the parts very freely. Secondly, one frequently found that no amount of traction upon the ends of the wires would retain the surfaces in accurate apposition after the grip of the lion forceps was relaxed.

Therefore I decided to treat the bones as one would the broken leg of a table or chair. The surfaces were brought into accurate apposition, and kept in their normal relationship by lion forceps. Holes were drilled above and below the forceps, and screws were driven in. The screws could be passed in any direction, and they retained the surfaces in an apposition more accurate and more forcible than I fancy can be attained by any other mechanical arrangement.

As far as I know, they cause no subsequent trouble; should they do so they can be removed through an incision equal to the diameter of the head of the screw.

Although I have limited myself to the consideration of the difficulties experienced in establishing exact continuity of the fragments in oblique fractures of the tibia and fibula, yet occasionally in a transverse fracture of the tibia it may be absolutely necessary to expose the broken ends before they can be brought into accurate apposition. As instances of this mode of treatment I am bringing three cases before the Society, as they were all done during the same take-in week, and represent the more simple and effectual means of approximation of the surfaces by screw pressure.

If the conclusions at which I have arrived are correct, it is obvious that any surgeon who resorts to the treatment of oblique fractures of both tibia and fibula, in labourers, by manipulation and splinting, without having previously explained to the patient the consequent disadvantages under which he will very possibly labour, and urged on him the importance of operative interference, is acting unjustly to his patient.

In the case of compound fractures of these bones it is equally advisable to procure perfect union, but for obvious reasons the surgeon is unable to offer the patient the same certainty of a successful result as he can when operating on a recent fracture.

Case 1—D. M., aet. 34, admitted under my care December 17, 1893. He fell with his leg twisted under him. The tibia was found to be fractured obliquely about two inches above the malleolus, and the fibula was broken about its centre. The lower fragment was displaced behind and outside the upper. Small fragments were felt. No amount of manipulation or traction served to bring the fragments into anything like accurate apposition. His permission for an operation not being obtained, a splint with a foot-piece everted at an angle equal to its fellow was applied.

On January 8, 1894, as no callus could be felt, and as there was definite deformity, operative measures were urged on him, and he consented.

The fracture in the tibia was exposed by an incision $4\frac{1}{2}$ inches long, when its direction was seen to be very oblique, running downwards, outwards, and backwards. Several small fragments of bone and muscle intervened between the ends of the bone.

Another effort to reduce the fragments by manipulation and traction was made, and the result was observed through the incision, when it was quite obvious that it could not have been effectual in this case in producing anything like apposition. The fragments of bone and muscle which intervened were removed, and after much difficulty the broken surfaces were brought into accurate apposition by means of lion forceps, and two screws were inserted. The temperature on one occasion after the operation rose to 99.2°.

Lane then described two further similar cases.

In none of these cases was there ever any sign of pus.

I am very much indebted to Mr. F. J. Steward, who obtained for me the details of forty cases of fracture of both bones of the leg taken indiscriminately from those treated in Guy's Hospital, and from various infirmaries. He started his investigations in an attitude antagonistic to the conclusions at which I had arrived, and this fact therefore renders his observations all the more reliable and valuable. From a consideration of the cases he collected he obtained the following deductions, which fully bear out the statements I have made in the early part of this paper.

DEDUCTIONS FROM CASES

In 40 cases of fractures of the tibia and fibula below the middle of the leg in men following various occupations, 19 or 48 per cent. suffered financially, owing either to inability to follow their former occupation or to earn as much as was earned at their original occupation; 15, or 38 per cent., suffered pain at the seat of injury; and 6, or 15 per cent., had pain in the ankle. and 4 of them had pain in the knee-joint; 12, or 30 per cent., suffered from insecurity in the limb, in nearly every case this insecurity being referred to the ankle-joint. In several of these cases the pain and insecurity in the ankle-joint was not noticed till a period varying from one to ten years had elapsed after the injury was received showing that slow changes took place in the ankle-joint in consequence of the alteration in the mechanical arrangements of the limb produced by the fracture.

In 23 cases of similar fractures in men following occupations, which necessitated heavy work and lifting of weights, 13, or 56 per cent., suffered financially owing to inability to do such heavy work; 12, or 52 per cent., had pain either at the seat of fracture or in the ankle- or knee-joint or in both; and 9, or 39 per cent., suffered from more or less insecurity in the whole limb, this last being in all cases the cause of the inability to follow their former laborious occupations.

3 OPERATIONS ON JOINTS

Arthroplasty

Of all formal orthopaedic reconstructive procedures, the construction of new, movable joints was one of the first suggested. As long ago as 1770, Charles White proposed excision of the head and neck of the femur, but did not carry it out except on cadavers (Chelius, 1847).

After this, priorities are difficult to elucidate; one school developed arthroplasty for fixed joint deformities, and the other, larger school excised infected or severely damaged bone in the vicinity of the joints, and accepted the movement that occurred as a bonus. The instigators of each school lived on opposite sides of the Atlantic.

In 1822, Anthony White excised a hip joint at the Westminster Hospital, London, for sepsis, and for five years afterwards the hip preserved good movement.

John Rhea Barton performed an intertrochanteric osteotomy of the femur in Philadelphia in 1825 for a fixed flexed hip, and succeeded in producing a pseudo-arthrosis.

Similar operations were carried out in small numbers, and in 1831 Syme published a little book summarising the indications for the procedure. Thirty years later, Hodge in the U.S.A. produced an excellent review but noted that the mortality from excision of the hip was about 50 per cent., though this compared with a mortality rate of nearly 100 per cent. for amputation at the level of the hip. This encouraged Hugh Owen Thomas and others to advocate conservative treatment for infective hip conditions as far as possible.

After these early attempts at arthroplasty, stiffness seems to have been the main problem; further advances dealt with new devices to keep the raw bone ends apart—Verneuil interposed muscle in 1860, and this remained popular, but surgeons tried fascia, skin, oil, rubber, celluloid, ivory and membranes, whose origins would satisfy any witch doctor. The Colonna capsular arthroplasty described in 1932, based on principles laid down by Hey Groves, is derived from this type of arthroplasty. Subsequently, distraction proved sufficient to prevent ankylosis in most circumstances, and Robert Jones in 1921 and Girdlestone in 1945, became the principal advocates of this.

Excision arthroplasty, whilst satisfactory from many points of view, does produce undesirable stability. Smith Petersen of Boston realised that if the joint was to retain stability a proper congrous mechanical bearing was needed. This was the very situation that was most likely to fuse solid. He therefore introduced his cup to serve as an interposition membrane. At first he looked upon it as a mould—to mould the fibrocartilage as it developed over the raw bone ends—and planned to remove the mould when it had served its purpose. He spent a long time finding a suitable material from which to form a mould; he started with glass in 1923, then used viscalloid, Pyrex, bakelite, and it was not until 1938 that he used vitallium. This became the arthroplasty of the 1940's.

In the fifties the Judet brothers—Robert and Jean—dominated the scene with a new idea; replacement arthroplasty. The first one was carried out in 1946, and their experience appeared in book form in 1952. Their choice of materials, acrylic, proved as unfortunate as Smith Petersen's choice of his earlier materials, but was forced on them because stainless steel and other metals were not available in France just after the war. The failures of the acrylic, and the difficulties with nearly horizontal stem paved the way for the development of the Austin Moore and Thompson prostheses with their stronger materials and better stem design. The relative softness of the head of the acrylic prosthesis had not revealed another potential difficulty of a replacement arthroplasty which has become apparent with metal prostheses —the acetabulum wears out in certain cases. Replacement of both the acetabulum and femoral head is a logical development now under trial.

Parallel to the developments in the formation of false joints and new joints have been other attempts to revitalise joints by means of osteotomies. Kirmission in 1894 suggested high femoral osteotomy for longstanding irreducible dislocation of the hip. Lorenz in 1919 treated this condition by femoral section at the level of the acetabulum and displaced the distal fragment into the acetabulum to form a new joint. Shanz in 1922 described a lower osteotomy with angulation at the osteotomy site so that the upper fragment lay parallel to the pelvic wall, acting as a slight support.

This type of operation found a new use in 1935 when McMurray and Malkin independently wrote up a small series of osteotomies for the deformities of osteoarthritis of the hip. The pain was relieved. Since then the operation has been performed with increasing frequency and degrees of sophistication. In some ways it is the ultimate in arthroplasty technique, as in some cases it appears to stimulate the joint to renew itself.

Excision Arthroplasty: Anthony White, 1822

The first successful excision of the head of the thigh-bone was performed in Westminster Hospital by Anthony White in April, 1822.

Case.—John West, when nine years old, slipped downstairs, and slightly hurt his left hip. After a few weeks, he was observed to limp in his gait, and complained of stiffness and pain in his groin; and subsequently he lost the power of locomotion, had the usual symptoms of disease in the hip-joint, and the head of the thigh-bone became displaced, and rested far back on the dorsum ilii. He suffered very acutely, and underwent the usual treatment of cupping, blistering, and every other method of local and constitutional treatment for many months, but without benefit, and after a time suppuration in the joint took place, which was evacuated from the front and upper part of the thigh. Temporary relief was thus obtained, but during two years a succession of similar abscesses formed around, and small portions of bone were frequently protruded through the sinuses which remained, and more especially, from those formed over the pubes. At the end of the third year, he was in the greatest possible state of emaciation, no longer suffering acute pain, but exhausted by the previous suffering, and by an overwhelming discharge from numerous apertures. The integuments over the displaced bone had become at various parts absorbed, and the bone at these points was readily found to be in a state of superficial caries. The knee had been long imbedded and immovably fixed on the inner side of the opposite thigh, and the right side on which he could alone lie, was cruelly galled with bedridden ulcerations. The formation of fresh abscesses had for some months ceased and further diseased processes were not apprehended. In the month of April, it was determined, in consultation with Travers, to remove the head of the bone; the circumstances of his health, with the exception of great emaciation, not forbidding it.

He made an incision, divided the bone 2 inches below the greater trochanter and removed the upper end of the femur. The leg now became straight, and John West was nursed on his back with his leg in bandages.

The wound quickly healed; the various sinuses soon ceased to discharge, and the health of the patient speedily improved. Within twelve months he enjoyed the most useful compensation for the loss of the original joint, had perfect flexion and extension of the thigh, and every other motion except for turning the knee outwards. The limb, of course, remained shorter, by as much as had been cut off from the top of the thigh-bone.

He died of phthisis five years after the operation and an opportunity was thus obtained to study the parts. The specimen was put in the museum of the Royal College of Surgeons, and showed a fibrous ankylosis.

Arthroplasty: 1825

On the Treatment of Anchylosis, by the Formation of Artificial Joints

A new operation, devised and executed

by J. Rhea Barton, M.D.

A Surgeon of the Pennsylvania Hospital

I beg leave to call the attention of my professional brethren to the following paper, believing that it contains some new views, in relation to a deformity and lameness, hitherto, I think, excluded from the surgeon's list of curable complaints, and one of the opprobria of our art; I allude to a *firm, bony anchylosis* of the human joints.

It is well known, that no such deformity can be established, until the original natural structure of a joint shall have undergone an entire change. The beautifully polished cartilages tipping the articulations, which, when supplied with synovia, admit of such perfect movements over their surfaces, must previously be absorbed, leaving only the two rough ends of the bones to unite, and become incorporated, and, as it were, one bone. It is not surprising, therefore, that we should not have bestowed upon such defects a second thought, in reference to a cure; since parts once gone, cannot in living matter be replaced, as they may be in machinery of human construction. The restoration, therefore, of a natural joint, once destroyed, being impossible, what has always been our course to persons thus afflicted? It has been, to apprise them of their *irreparable* loss; leaving time only to reconcile them to a misfortune, entailed on them through after life. Having witnessed, about sixteen months ago, a most distressing instance of deformity and lameness, from an injury of the hip joint, it aroused me to much reflection on this subject, that eventuated in my adopting views, and a course of practice, which shall hereafter be detailed. I will relate the case referred to.

John Coyle, native of Philadelphia, twenty-one years of age, sailor on board the schr. Topaz, Captain Schyler, states, that on the 17th day of March, 1825, he fell from the hatchway into the ship's hold, upon the end of a barrel, a distance of about six or seven feet; that the force of the fall was sustained on the out side of his right hip; violent pain was the immediate consequence, and much tumefaction ensued; that after the injury, he arose with difficulty, and attempted to walk, thinks he made one or two steps, but was compelled to retire to his hammock, where he laid contracted for the space of about eighteen days; was then taken into Porto Cavello, and conveyed to the hospital. When lodged upon his bed, he placed himself on his side, with the injured limb uppermost, drawing the thigh to a right angle with the axis of the pelvis, and the knee resting on the sound side. In this posture he continued, without any material alteration, for the space of about five months; in the meantime, enduring all the suffering attendant upon a high degree of inflammation of one of the largest joints in the human body, and unalleviated by the support of splints, or a judicious antiphlogistic course of treatment. As might naturally be expected, a rigid and deformed limb was the result of such disease, combatted only by the administration of some simple liniment.

With regard to the real nature of the primary injury sustained, little can be said. The opinion on this point, of the medical attendant, under whose special care the patient was placed in the hospital, is not known. Dr. Murphy, surgeon general, who occasionally saw him, believed it to be a dislocation. On board of the Topaz, previous to his removal to the hospital, two physicians, belonging respectively to an English and French vessel of war, laying in port, inspected the limb, in company with the American Consul, Dr. Litchfield. Two of these gentlemen thought there was fracture; the French physician believed it to be some form of luxation. It is certain therefore, from the difference of sentiment, that there was much obscurity in the case.

In October, 1825, Coyle returned to Philadelphia, having been sent home by our Consul.

Early on his arrival, he exhibited himself to me. He was then supported by crutches, having the thigh drawn up nearly to a right angle with the axis of the pelvis, and the knee turned inward, and projecting over the sound thigh; so that the outside of the foot presented forward. There was considerable enlargement round the hip, which so much obscured the case, even at this date, as to prevent me from forming any positive opinion as to the real nature of the original injury. From the fixed and immovable condition of the limb, it was impossible to ascertain whether, in a straight position, there would be shortening, and, if any, to what extent. The general feature of the limb bore somewhat the resemblance of that resulting from a dislocation into the ischiatic notch; yet the position in which the great trochanter stood, in relation to the superior anterior spinous process, discouraged such a belief. All things considered, I was rather inclined to the opinion, that there had been neither fracture nor luxation; but that the violence of the fall had produced an extensive contusion of the round ligament and joint, and that disorganisation had followed the consequent inflammation. On this point, whatever might have been the nature of the accident, I thought I might feel assured, that *now* all articular movement was gone, and that true anchylosis had taken place. Trusting, however, to the fallibility of my judgment, and wishing, for the patient's sake, that it might prove erroneous, I was induced to admit him into the Pennsylvania Hospital, with the view of employing extension on the limb for some weeks, in hopes that its malposition might thereby be corrected. A perseverance, however, in this treatment, only proved the unalterable state of the hip-joint, and confirmed my early formed opinion. He subsequently fell under the care of my estimable friends and colleagues, Drs. Hewson and Parrish, in their respective tours of surgical attendance in the hospital, where we several times considered his case in consultation, and were united in our final decision, that any further attempt to release the joint would be useless.

Finding Coyle still in the hospital, a year after his admission, much reflection on his case led me to propose to my colleagues, the following operation, viz. to make an incision through the integuments, of six or seven inches in length, one half extending above, and the other below, the great trochanter; this to be met by a transverse section, of four or five inches in extent; the two forming a crucial incision, the four angles of which were to meet opposite to the most prominent point of the great trochanter; then to detach the fascia, and, by turning the blade of the scalpel sideways, to separate anteriorly all muscular structure from the bone, without unnecessarily dividing their fibres. Having done this, in like manner, behind and between the two trochanters, to divide the bone transversely through the great trochanter, and part of the neck of the bone, by means of a strong and narrow saw, made for the purpose; this being accomplished, to extend the limb, and dress the wound. After the irritation from the operation shall have passed away, to prevent, if possible, by gentle and daily movement of the limb, etc., the formation of bony union; and to establish an attachment by ligament only, as in cases of ununited fractures, or artificial joints, as they are called.

In this proposition, four material points presented themselves for consideration, viz. the practicability of the operation; the degree of risk to life, consequent thereto; the probability of being able to arrest ossific re-union; and the reasonable prospect of benefiting the patient thereby. The arguments I adduced in favour of such an operation, were these: that the anatomy of the part did not present any insurmountable obstacle to it. The fear of cutting into a joint was not to be entertained here, since, from previous disease, all the characteristics of a joint were gone; synovial membrane destroyed; cartilages absorbed; and an amalgamation of the head of the femur with the acetabulum, had taken place. That the shock to the vital system would not, probably, be greater than is frequently endured from accidental injuries, and other operations. That, if the opinion commonly assigned as the cause of the formation of false joints, after fractures, be true, such as frequent motion in the broken ends of the bone, a deficiency of tone in the system, etc., these agents could be resorted to with promising results.

In order to decide the important question, as to the benefit which the patient might be reasonably expected to derive from such an operation, it was necessary to consider how nearly a joint, thus artificially formed, would resemble, in its construction and functions, the natural articulation. What change the divided ends of the bone would undergo; whence would be derived its cartilaginous surfaces, its ligaments, its capsule, and its synovia; and, finally, what was to restrain its undue motions. My hopes of improving his condition, were founded upon the following facts and observations in relation to these points. That a bone, once divided, in a person otherwise healthy, must again unite, either by bone or by ligament; no case, to my knowledge, being on record, where a broken bone remained always afterward destitute of attachment between the divided extremities; except in cases where one of the fragments has been so small, or so scantily supplied with blood, as to be unable to contribute its part in the restorative process, being sufficiently vascular only to retain its own vitality, as in case of the separation of the head of a bone. If, therefore, ossific union should be arrested, ligamentous adhesions would maintain the connexion. Writers observe, and it is confirmed by my own experience, that when a fracture does not become consolidated, in the course of time, the rugged edges are removed by absorption; the separated ends become condensed, smooth, and polished, and tipped with a kind of cartilaginous substance; they are likewise inclosed within a sort of capsule. Observation has also proved to me, that this ligamentous structure, formed around and connecting the ends of an old fracture, is possessed of great strength; so much so, that I have, in several instances, witnessed persons sustaining the entire weight of their bodies on the ligaments of a false joint, requiring only lateral support to the limb. The freedom and latitude of motion, in such cases, and total insensibility to pain, after a sufficient lapse of time, I had also witnessed, and were encouraging arguments. In the operation here proposed, no such great strength of ligaments as will support the body, would be required; since, from the *transverse* section of the trochanter, bone will rest against bone, and strength in them sufficient only to prevent dislocation, would be necessary. From my inquiries into the manner in which this joint was to be lubricated, I did not expect that a synovial membrane and fluid, in all their characters, would be generated; but ample proofs were not wanting, of the immediate resources of nature in defending parts from injurious friction, in whatever point of the body it might be required, either by an exhalation from the adjacent structure, or by the intervention of a bursa. In the common false joint, where motion is discouraged as much as possible, sufficient moisture is there exuded to prevent painful attrition. It might reasonably be expected, therefore, that where motion was continual, the lubricating moisture would be more abundantly exhaled. In un-united fractures, the false joint is uncontrollable, because there are no muscles specially adapted for its restraint; but in the joint thus to be formed, *the will* alone must influence its movements; since nearly all of the muscles which exercised their control over the original joint, would be carefully preserved, to have a similar power over this; which is, in fact, a mere transfer of the point of articulation and resistance, from the head of the bone in the acetabulum, to the upper end of the shaft of the femur, against the great trochanter.

Although I did not think it essential to the melioration of my patient's condition, that the ends of the bone should at its section undergo any change, further than by the absorption of the asperities, I did believe, that nature would not passively witness my labours to effect what she has herself so often endeavoured, unaided by art, to accomplish; but that she would be ready to co-operate with me, and to extend to completion, that which human art alone would be incapable of—the formation of a new and useful joint, as a substitute for that which disease had annihilated, either by the conversion of the trochanter into a socket. or by some more wise design. Dissections of old luxations, and of fractures, near joints, present many ingenious and wonderful alteration of original, and depositions of new structure, to restore the functions and uses of parts impaired by accidents and disease. All authors notice these attempts at restoration Sir Astley Cooper, in his "Treatise on Dislocations and

Fractures of the Joints," has particularly mentioned them, and given many interesting plates, illustrative of nature's unassisted achievements. Such circumstances strongly encouraged me in the experiment, and were considered as auguries of a favourable result.

These views were fully explained to my colleagues, and were accompanied by the assurance, that my patient had been fairly apprised of his present condition, and of the nature and intentions of the operation proposed; that he had not merely acceded to it, but that, after placing his sufferings, the difficulties, risks to life, the chances of failure, and the dangers eventually of aggravated lameness, in the strongest and most exaggerated light, he had expressed his willingness to endure any pain, or duration of suffering, and to subject himself to all hazards, for the remotest prospect of relief.

Accordingly, on the 22nd day of November, 1826, assisted by Drs. Hewson and Parrish, I proceeded to the operation publicly in the Pennsylvania Hospital.

To a large medical class, and many respectable physicians, assembled, I again represented the nature of the case, and of the operation, and the views and course of reasoning which induced me to adopt it, stating likewise, that I wished it to be distinctly understood, that a submission to my contemplated plans had not been urged upon my patient by any false or delusory promises; but that an explanation of his existing condition, and of the means proposed to be attempted for his relief, were fully made to him, in language adapted to his right comprehension of the matter, as well as by my colleagues, as by myself; and that he had authorised me thus publicly to state, that he was prepared to assume all and the exclusive responsibility for the issue.

With this exculpation, therefore, the operation, as already detailed, was put into effect. The integuments and fascia being divided and raised, the muscles in contact with the bone, around part of the great trochanter, were carefully detached, and a passage thereby made, just large enough to admit of the insinuation of my fore-fingers, before and behind the bone; the tips of which now met around the lower part of the cervix of the femur, a little above its root. The saw was readily applied, and, without any difficulty, a separation of the bone was effected. The thigh was now released, and I immediately turned out the knee, extended the leg, and placed the limbs side by side; by a comparison of which, in reference to length, the unsound member betrayed a shortening of about half an inch. This might have been caused partly by a distortion of the pelvis. Not one blood-vessel required to be secured. Union by the first intention was not attempted; the lips of the wound were only supported by adhesive plaster and slight dressings. The patient was put to bed, and Dr. Sault's splints were applied, to support the limb.

The operation, though severe, was not of long duration, it being accomplished in the space of about seven minutes.

Postoperatively, the patient kept the leg still for nearly six weeks, and then began to move it in bed. By nine weeks the wound was soundly healed and he stood out of bed on crutches. A few days later he took a few steps and developed good control over the false joint.

Ten years later Barton gives a follow up report about him.

> The patient, upon whom this operation was performed, enjoyed the use of his artificial joint for six years; during which period he pursued a business (trunk-making) with great industry, earning for himself a comfortable subsistence, and a small annual surplus.

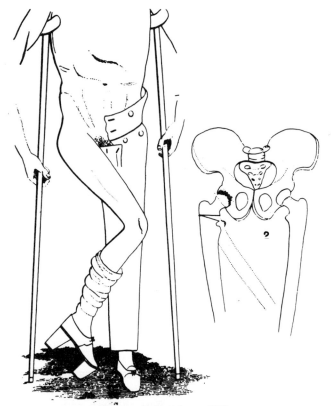

Barton: Arthroplasty of Hip

Pecuniary losses however, through the reverses of those in whose hands he had confided his means, sunk him into a state of despondency and desperation, followed by habits of intemperance. This, with all its train of evils, abuse of health, etc, was, no doubt, the cause of the change which afterwards took place in the artificial joint. It gradually became more and more rigid, and finally, all motion ceased in the part. With this exception, the benefits of my operation were retained and fully appreciated until the period of his death; for as the limb had been freed from deformity and restored to a useful position, he had no occasion even for a cane to aid in walking. During an attack of the Asiatic cholera, he expressed a desire that I should be sent for, in order that he might renew his bequest to me of the parts interested in the operation. He recovered from the cholera, but subsequently died of phthisis pulmonalis. The autopsy exhibited the parts as described in the published case, but with the artificial joint ancholysed; a change which had been effected within the two years previous to his death. With ordinary care, in all probability, this would not have taken place.

The final history of this case presents now the important fact, that benefit had resulted, which fully requited the individual for the pains he had endured, and were considered by him, even after the closure of the joint, yet an ample reward for the operation he had undergone.

In the original article he goes on to explore the possibilities of arthroplasty.

Having now established the fact, that an artificial joint can be substituted for the loss of the natural articulation at the hip, it becomes a matter of importance to ascertain how far the same principles are applicable to the formation of new joints in other parts of the body, where natural motion has been lost. My reflections on the point, have not presented any forbidding circumstances; but it is not in every joint, that the loss of motion would be sufficiently important to call for the aid of a painful operation. The most serious evil is sustained by the loss of the hip, knee, shoulder, elbow, great toe, and finger joints, and of the lower jaw, and these, I believe, may all come within the reach of amendment by operation, if the muscles which move these respective joints are in a sound and efficient state. If they have been lost, it would be palpably wrong to form a joint, since its unrestrained motion would be more troublesome than a rigid limb. A transverse section of the bones would be proper, if the operation were to be attempted at the shoulder, knee, fingers, or toes; but an angular division would be necessary at the elbow, in order to preserve some resemblance to the natural joint at this part.

I hope I will not be understood as entertaining the belief, that this treatment will be applicable to, and judicious in, every case of anchylosis. I believe the operation would be justifiable *only* under the following circumstances, viz., where the patient's general health is good, and his constitution sufficiently strong; where the rigidity is not confined to the soft parts, but is actually occasioned by a consolidation of the joint; where all the muscles and tendons, that were essential to the ordinary movements of the former joint, are sound, and not incorporated by firm adhesions with the adjacent structure; where the disease, causing the deformity, has entirely subsided; where the operation can be performed through the original point of motion, or so near to it, that the use of most of the tendons and muscles will not be lost; and, finally, where the deformity, or inconvenience, is such, as will induce the patient to endure the pain, and incur the risks of an operation.

James Syme, 1799-1870

James Syme was born in Princes Street, Edinburgh, the son of a lawyer. Whilst a student at Edinburgh University he found a way of dissolving rubber and discovered that when this was applied to material it became water-proof. Had he realised the commercial value of this, his name, and not that of Mackintosh, would have been attached to this product.

After qualifying, he opened a school of anatomy and later a very successful private clinic. For a short while he was Professor of Surgery at University College Hospital. He found it difficult to get on the staff of the hospital at Edinburgh; however, the Professor of Surgery eventually agreed to retire at the age of 81 on the condition that his successor paid him a pension. Syme acquiesced and obtained hospital beds. Later Lister became his assistant and married his daughter.

Syme is remembered for the introduction of conservative alternatives to major amputations. In 1831 he published a booklet on joint excision as an alternative to amputation for grossly diseased joints. His opening paragraphs could be used unchanged today for a paper dealing with prosthetic replacement of joints. Later, joint excision fell into disrepute because it tended to supplant all other methods of treatment for tuberculous joints and the succeeding generation of surgeons decried it in favour of rest. He introduced his amputation in 1844 as an alternative to below knee amputation which was then the standard level.

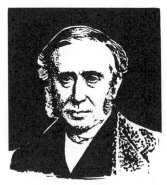

On the Diseases and Injuries of the Joints in which Excision may be Performed: James Syme, 1831

Owing to the improvements of modern surgery, more particularly in the treatment of aneurysms, fractures and necrosis, amputation of the extremities is now very seldom performed in civil practice except in cases of disease or injury of the joints.

Though amputation is a measure very disagreeable both to the patient and to the surgeon, it has hitherto, with hardly any exception, been regarded as the only safe and efficient means of removing diseased joints which do not admit recovery. The idea of cutting out merely the morbid parts and leaving the sound portion of the limb, seems to have hardly ever occurred, or to have met with so many objections that it was almost instantly abandoned.

Arthroplasty of the Great Toe: John Neville Davies-Colley, 1843-1900

The son of a physician at Chester, Davies-Colley trained at Guy's and became Assistant Surgeon to the hospital four years after qualifying. He married the daughter of the Treasurer of Guy's (who had a powerful influence at the Selection Board), before being elected to the staff. It is said that his predecessor had been engaged to the Treasurer's daughter, but on being appointed to the staff broke the engagement off.

He was a good lecturer and a bold surgeon by all accounts.

Although it is widely stated by some of our more patriotic surgeons that he antedated Keller, this does not seem to be so. He described and treated hallux rigidus by removing the base of the proximal phalanx—he did not touch the exostosis. Steele, in the States, described in 1898 the same operation as Davies-Colley for relief of severe hallux valgus.

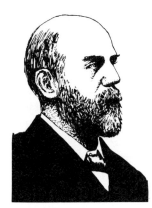

On Contraction of the Metatarso-phalangeal Joint of the Great Toe (Hallux flexus). With Cases

by N. Davies-Colley, 1887

Having now for many years been familiar with a painful deformity of the foot which appears to have escaped the notice of our surgical writers, I venture to bring before the Society a short account of five cases which have been under my care. The disease consists simply of the flexion of the first phalanx of the great toe through an angle of from 30° to 60° upon the first metatarsal bone. There is no ankylosis, but the phalanx cannot be extended, and the attempt to execute this movement by external force gives rise to considerable pain. The metatarso-phalangeal joint is usually somewhat enlarged and thickened. There is no deviation of the first phalanx outwards, as in the common affection called hallux valgus. Walking is very painful and difficult, and the patient is obliged to bear his weight as much as possible upon the outer border of the foot. The phalangeal joint is healthy, and the ungual phalanx is maintained in a straight line with the first.

There are two causes which I have been able to assign to this condition, viz.: (1) A blow, setting up some inflammation in the metatarsal-phalangeal point; and (2) ill-fitting and unyielding boots, especially in individuals in whom the first toe is much longer, and therefore in advance of, the other toes. In the former class of cases, I suppose that during the rest following an injury the toe becomes flexed, in order to relieve the painful tension of the swollen joint, much in the same way as the knee-joint is affected by a similar condition. By the time that the more acute symptoms have subsided the short fleshy muscles of the sole have contracted, and adhesions have formed, which prevent the restoration of the normal position of the joint. In the latter class it is easy to understand that the constant backward pressure of a short strong boot upon the tip of the great toe must lead to some deviation from its ordinary form. If this deviation be outwards hallux valgus is produced, but if the toe be forced directly backwards, flexion takes place at the metatarso-phalangeal joint; a projecting angle is formed on the dorsal aspect of the joint, and the pressure of the rigid upper leather upon this projection causes inflammation, which fixes the bones in their new position. When once a pronounced deviation of this kind has been produced the flexor muscles act with greater advantage, and tend to increase the deformity. All my five cases have been in young men. I suppose it affects the male sex because men have more walking to do, are more liable to injury and wear stiffer boots. I am in some doubt as to why I have met no well-marked cases in older men, but I am inclined to think that in later life the great toe may leave its position of direct flexion and the condition may change to that of hallux valgus. . . .

Case 4. Hallux flexus; resection of proximal half of first phalanx; cure.

William J., aet. 21, painter, was admitted under my care into Luke ward, Guy's Hospital, on February 11, 1885, suffering from flexion of first phalanx of the left great toe through 45°. He had had it for three years and could assign no cause. It began with pain in the joint and occasional shooting pain up the leg. At the same time he noticed that the skin over the joint was red. He was not aware that he had worn a tight boot. Walking was difficult and painful. He could use the extensor proprius hallucis well, and no band could be felt on the inner side of the sole. Abductors and adductors were not-affected, and he could slightly flex and extend the toe. There was a little prominence of the metatarso-phalangeal joint of the right great toe on the dorsum, but no marked flexion of the phalanx.

On a subsequent occasion I found that the right great toe was so abnormally long that it projected three-eighths to half an inch in front of the tip of the second toe.

On February 13, I excised the proximal half of the first phalanx under ether, by an incision one and a half inches long at the junction of the upper and inner surface of the joint. The articular cartilage was a little worn and fibrous, but there was no other evidence of disease in the joint.

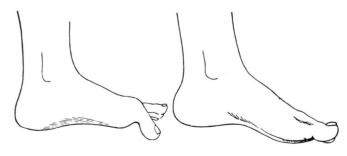

Davies-Colley: Hallux Flexus

By March 5 the wound had healed by primary union. By the 30th he could walk well on the flat foot.

Twenty-two months after the operation he came to show himself, and my late dresser, Mr. Fisher, made a drawing of his foot. The first phalanx was in a line with the metatarsal bone. The joint was stiff but not ankylosed, the range of passive movement being 5° to 10°. The scar of the operation was smooth, and difficult to recognise, and there was nothing abnormal about the appearance of the foot.

The only pain he had in the joint was when he put on his boots. The day before I saw him he had walked twenty miles without any discomfort.

Colonel William Keller, 1874-1959

Keller introduced his operation for bunions at the very beginning of his surgical career, whilst he was working in Manila during the Philippine insurrection. Though it is now one of the most commonly performed operations, he was not very interested in it, but went on to achieve fame in the field of general surgery, and in particular in the field of pulmonary surgery in its early days.

He was born in Connecticut in 1874, and graduated from Virginia in 1899. The following year he became a contract surgeon with the U.S. Army, and was commissioned in 1902. He moved around hospitals in the U.S.A. and the Pacific until the First World War when he was assigned to the American Expeditionary Forces as Director of Professional Services.

In 1919 he joined the Walter Reed Hospital to head the Department of Surgery. During this time he developed an unroofing technique for empyema, a type of inguinal hernia repair, a repair for recurrent shoulder dislocations (cruciate implication of the inferior capsule through an axillary approach), and the tunnel skin graft. This last was rather intriguing; when an ulcer or scar was to be grafted, he made a tunnel underneath it and laid the graft in it. The roof kept the graft in position and the roof either disappeared by itself or could be removed.

He was offered the post of Surgeon General but refused because he wanted to continue clinical surgery. He remained at the Walter Reed until his retirement in 1935. He was one of those fortunate people who only need four hours' sleep a night, and so have more time to work than most. On his retirement, he was, by special Congressional legislation, made a consultant with pay and allowances for life, the first man to be so honoured in U.S. Army history. In 1953 an annual lecture was named after him.

Keller's Operation: 1904

The writer uses an operation which eliminates all interference with the tripod of the foot or its normal level. It is based upon deductions made as to the common cause of the unsatisfactory results following operations heretofore employed; while the number of operations

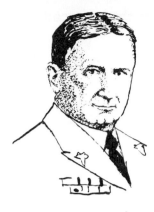

which have been performed by this method is limited, he feels most confident that the satisfactory results in the cases reported will invariably follow the operation, if properly performed in every case.

Operation.—A longitudinal incision, two inches in length, is made along the inner side of the foot, exposing the first metatarsophalangeal articulation. The skin and tissues over the head of the metatarsal bone are retracted; the joint is then opened and opposing articular ends are separated; the periosteal covering over the lateral enlargement and adjoining part of bone are pushed back; and the exostosis with about one-eighth on an inch of the bone is removed by rongeur forceps or preferably, with a small saw. The tendon of the flexor longus hallucis is freed by blunt dissection from the under surface of the base of the first phalanx, sufficiently to pass a Gigli saw around the bone; the periosteum is pushed back, disarticulation accomplished, and the articular head of the first phalanx is removed. Particular care should be taken throughout the operation to protect the periosteum from needless destruction, and an effort should be made to preserve enough of it to cover the exposed surface of the bone.

A small gauze drain is inserted between the head of the metatarsal bone and the sawed end of the phalanx (this drain is removed after forty-eight hours). The wound is carefully sutured; the toe being maintained at normal extension by a narrow internal lateral splint. Passive motion is begun on the fifth day.

Cases reported below are evidences of the more satisfactory results to be obtained from the operative method advocated.

Miss ——, trained nurse, had suffered from bunions on both feet or nine years, and had not worn leather shoes for several years. One week before the operation the pain became so excruciating that she had to abandon her duties as nurse.

Operation as described. The recovery was uncomplicated and the patient resumed her duties after three weeks. Up to this time (six months after the operation), not the slightest discomfort has been felt.

The advantages of the operation are as follows: First: The normal tripod of the foot is not disturbed. Second: The danger of ankylosis is comparatively slight. Third: it can be used when the normal arch of the foot is high, while the old operation can be done with safety only when the deformity is complicated by flat foot.

In a second paper eight years later, Keller reported the results of 26 operations, which seems a very slow rate of accumulation, and suggests some modifications of technique. He adopted an eyebrow incision and removed more exostosis. "The cut is obliquely upward and outward along the length of the metatarsal. This cut extends from the inner edge of the sesamoid below, to a line above, which is well past the middle of the dorsum of the bone." Soft tissue was interposed between the bone ends, as shown in the diagram.

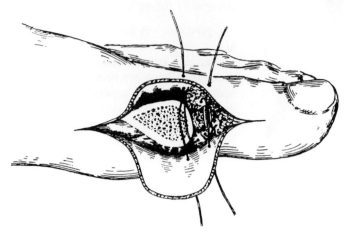

Keller's operation. Primary incision exposing the first metatarso-phalangeal joint, showing also the sutures.

Arthrodesis

Perhaps the first person to carry out an arthrodesis for deformity was Henry Park in Liverpool in 1781. The son of an apothecary in Liverpool, he was apprenticed to Pott, to whom he dedicated the technique. Apart from describing arthrodesis, his other chief claim to fame is that he delivered Gladstone.

It was exactly 100 years later that Albert of Vienna suggested arthrodesis as a means of treating flail limbs.

An Account of a New Method of Treating Diseases of the Joints of the Knee and Elbow in a Letter to Mr. Percivall Pott by H. Park of Liverpool. 1781

Joint infections all too often ended in amputations; he thought that there were other untried surgical resources that would produce a better result.

> The resource I mean is the *total extirpation of the articulation*, or the entire removal of the extremities of all the bones which form the joints, with the whole, or as much as possible, of the Capsular ligament; thereby obtaining a cure by means of Callus or by uniting the femur and tibia, when practised on the knee; and the Humerus, Radius and Ulna, when at the elbow, into one bone, without any movable articulation.
>
> The practicability of such an operation, with a probability of success, occurred to me some years ago; but as the undertaking appeared liable to many difficulties and objections, I wished to avoid being too precipitate in the attempt, and therefore frequently made it a subject of conversation with different Gentlemen of the Profession. The principal difficulties that occurred, either from my

own reflections, or the observations of my friends were as follows, viz.: the hazard of wounding the principal blood vessels; the great inflammation and large suppurations usually consequent on wounds of the articulations; the uncertainty of obtaining a firm Callus; the loss of the insertions of the extensor muscles; the doubt respecting the utility of the limb, provided a cure could be obtained; the uncertainty of removing the whole disease when caries gave rise to operation; and, when undertaken on account of a scrophulous affection of the joints, the hazard of return of the same disease.

These difficulties he considered and finally discounted after rehearsing the procedure on cadavers. He decided to put the operation into practice.

I had under my care in the Infirmary, Hector M'Caghen, a strong, robust, Scotch sailor, aged 33, who was admitted for a diseased knee of ten years standing; the joint, though pretty considerably enlarged, was by no means so much so as is frequently met with in scrophulous affections; yet the integuments were so tense as to appear incapable of further distension; the contraction of the Flexor Muscles was such as to draw back the leg, so as to form a right angle with the thigh, in which position it was immovably fixed; apparently some degree of union had begun to take place, but this could not yet be determined with certainty, as every attempt to communicate to the joint the smallest amount of motion, gave him the most excruciating pain.

Conservative treatment did not help, and the patient's pain led him to request amputation. Park suggested his operation, and carried it out on 2nd July, 1781. He made a cruciate incision, removed the patella, and sawed off 2 inches of femur and 1 inch of tibia, making transverse cuts. This was just enough to allow the sawn ends of the bones to lie in close contact, held by the contracted hamstrings. He inserted a few skin sutures, a minimum of dressings, and placed the leg in a case of tin.

The wound discharged profusely for some time and did not heal for about three months. He started to go about on crutches, and by five months after the operation union was strong enough for him to lift the leg up straight, and in another month it felt solid. He subsequently had 3 inches shortening, and wore a raised shoe and a protective leather support. Hugh M'Caghen returned to sea once more with a leg that felt strong. (In the same letter Park describes an arthrodesis of elbow.)

Syme gives a little more of the history of Hugh M'Caghen. He continued as a sailor and was shipwrecked twice without his leg causing any trouble and finally drowned in the Mersey when a boat overturned.

Eduard Albert, 1841-1900

Albert was born in Bohemia, and studied in Vienna. He became Professor of Surgery at Innsbruck in 1873 and later transferred to Vienna. An excellent teacher and man of ideas, he described arthrodesis to improve function of flail limbs, synovectomy, the transplantation of nerves, sciatic scoliosis and Achilles bursitis.

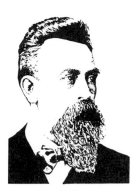

Some Cases of Artificially Produced Ankyloses in Paralysed Limbs: E. Albert, 1881

I have tried the idea of making paralysed legs, especially those incapable of bearing weight due to poliomyelitis, more useable and more independent of appliances by artificial ankylosis in the following cases and found it successful:

1. Josef F. aged 22; admitted 20 July 1881. Left leg, especially calf, grossly wasted. Muscles of hip joint functioning perfectly. Knee and foot completely flail; foot in slight equinus. This leg which was attacked by poliomyelitis in childhood is notably shorter.

20 July. Resection of the knee joint through Volkmann's incision and division of the patella. Removal of the capsule. Enough cut off the femur to allow the level of section to pass through the fossa inter-condyloideus; a thin disc cut off the tibia. Two bone sutures between femur and tibia, and one between the two halves of the patella. Sutures, drainage, Lister bandage, and splint fixation.

The wound healed mostly per primam, but in a few places with some sepsis.

2 September. Erysipelas was in the wound.

11 September. Abscess opened below tuberosity. Erysipelas faded.

15 October. Firm joint confirmed.

2 November. Silver wires removed; joint solid and immoveable.

After the patient had walked around for some time on crutches, he was, at the end of November, given a support which was fixed to the unstable foot by means of a lace up boot and two side irons. The irons pass above the knee so as to protect the rigid knee joint from accidental injury for some time. At discharge on 12th December the knee is completely ankylosed.

2. *Another knee fusion. Successful.*

3. *Another knee fusion. Some movement remained.*

4. Therese W. Aged 11. Struck down by poliomyelitis aged $1\frac{1}{2}$ years. Left leg almost 3 cm short, wasted. Calf much more wasted than the thigh. Hip and knee joint normally actively mobile. Foot in fixed equino-varus position. Pronounced hump on the dorsum of the foot. Toes capable of active flexion and the existing plantar flexion could be increased. The dorsal group of muscles paralysed. The foot completely unstable, walking difficult.

29 December, 1881. Achilles tenotomy, then the ankle joint opened up through a dorsal incision which also divided the attenuated tendons of the toe extensors. The cartilage covering the talus and the articular surface of the fibula removed. The cartilage was extraordinarily easy to peel off, as is almost always the case with paralysed extremities. Wound sutured, Lister bandage, Plaster cast.

On the sixteenth day erysipelas spreading only over the calf and disappearing by the 23rd day. In order to relieve the equinus deformity of the foot and to ankylose it in the neutral position of the ankle joint the plaster cast had to be removed several times and replaced after further correction. When the last cast was applied it appeared that slight overcorrection had been produced so that a minor degree of pes calcaneus seemed to have developed. In order to achieve better control, the leg was fixed to a splint, of which the longer part was fixed to the calf and the shorter to the foot, fixing the two at right angles. After 6 weeks the patient could put her weight on the foot. She was discharged 9 weeks after operation; the talus and lower leg were firmly united; the foot was in a position of very slight pronation; in walking the leg moved in one piece, but the foot was no longer unstable and the patient was plantigrade. She was given a supporting appliance (a lace up shoe with a side iron).

The cases I report can only be regarded as encouraging; the expected results were achieved, in fact one might say that the results exceeded expectation since one might have doubted whether bone might be expected to fuse in a paralysed leg.

But nor should these cases be considered more than encouraging; only further experience can show how one should plan the operative technique and how applicable this method is to other joints.

4 OPERATIONS ON TENDONS

The ancients are said to have repaired tendons and nerves, but as they did not distinguish between these structures until the Renaissance, information is a little uncertain.

In the seventeenth century tenotomy began to be practised in Holland. Isaac Minnius performed a tenotomy for torticollis in 1685. A hundred years later Lorenz of Frankfurt treated a clubfoot by division of the tendo Achillis. Delpeche of Montpellier repeated this on several occasions between 1816 and 1823, but gave it up because of complications leaving it to Stromeyer to popularise it from 1831 onwards. It was brought to England, as will be described, by Little, and was soon to be used for a range of fixed deformities—even for squint.

Myotomy came into vogue soon afterwards but floundered after a period of trial on the posterior vertebral muscles in the treatment of scoliosis.

Tendon grafting and tendon transplantation are described below by Waterman, who himself made many contributions to the field.

Tenotomy

Little on Clubfoot and its Treatment by Tenotomy: 1839

The term club-foot has been indiscriminately applied to three kinds of deformity, to which surgical writers have affixed the term *varus*, *valgus*, and *pes equinus*; and the ordinary laconic description of their symptoms has not usually extended further than stating, that in varus the toe of the affected limb is twisted inwards, so that the patient walks more or less upon the outer ankle; that valgus is the contrary deformity, the toe being turned outwards, and the patient compelled to tread upon the inner ankle; and that the pes equinus is that state of the foot in which the individual rests the weight of the body upon the toes only.

So long as a foot, altered in its form according to any of these different types, was looked upon as a shapeless mass, an organ deficient perhaps in some of its parts, and requiring for restoration to a more natural figure, to be merely moulded and compressed by mechanical instruments for a considerable length of time (the case being considered incurable if these means did not succeed), that brief definition of symptoms, and the nomenclature commonly used, appeared sufficient. But as chirurgical means of overcoming these deformities have been discovered, a more strict description of their symptoms is necessary to distinguish the cases which are fitted for operation from those which are curable without an operation, or from others which are incurable by any means. The nomenclature, for the same reason, has appeared to me to require some additions; the causes and varieties of deformities of the feet being numerous, the three names, varus, valgus, and equinus, are insufficient to designate them. I have therefore proposed to employ the classical word *Talipes* (hitherto applied to one species only), as a generic term, to include all those deformities of the feet produced, as will be seen, by contraction of certain muscles, to restrict it to deformities from this source; and to use the terms varus, valgus, and equinus, to designate the specific forms of these diseases.

A description of the forms of clubfoot follows. One may judge that many of his cases were the result of poliomyelitis, as wasting of the thigh and shortening of the leg were frequent accompaniments of the deformity. After discussing pathology, he describes treatment under the headings of medical treatment (antispasmodics), splintage, and tenotomy.

There are many cases both of congenital and non-congenital Talipes in which the medical part of the plan is unnecessary, either in consequence of the paralytic or spasmodic cause having subsided, or from having existed too great a length of time to render removal probable, and where there remains only an inconsiderable *structural* shortening, although accompanied with great deformity. These cases may be cured in the space of a few months, without relapse, by means of mechanical treatment alone . . . to prevent the muscles from becoming affected with structural or organic shortening, through remaining a long period in a contracted state, more particularly during the earliest period of life, when the growth of parts is very rapid, manipulation, friction, and the use of mechanical apparatus, properly contrived and adjusted, must be resorted to. I have by this method of proceeding cured, without operation, cases which had been presented to me for relief by this *dernier ressort* of our art.

If, however, either in congenital cases, in consequence of the affection of the muscles having occurred at an early period of foetal existence; or in non-congenital cases, from the deformity having continued unchecked for too great length of time—structural shortening of the contracted muscles have taken place, which is usually ascertained by the inelastic rigid nature of the contraction of the muscles, the tendons of those muscles which resist the restoration of the foot to its proper form, must, provided that there be no accidental displacement or deformity of the bones, or ankylosis, be divided by the knife, in order to obtain a cure.

In most cases of Talipes equinus, and in many of T. varus, which require an operation, the tendo Achillis only is required to be divided; in other cases of Talipes equinus I have sometimes found it necessary likewise to divide the tendons of the tibialis posticus and flexor longus pollicis muscles. In severe long-standing cases of Talipes varus the section of the tendons of the anterior tibial, posterior tibial, extensor proprius and flexor longus pollicis muscles is requisite, in addition to division of the tendo Achillis, in order to facilitate the restoration of the foot to its natural shape and position. The case of congenital Talipes valgus already mentioned will indicate the parts which it may be found necessary to divide in that form of disease.

As I regard Stromeyer to be the regenerator of this important addition to our means of curing club-foot, with other contractions of the ankle, and similar deformities of various parts of the body, and having experienced in my own person the success of his method of treatment, corroborated by the numerous cases which I have cured by the same means, I shall here only briefly enumerate the principles recommended by Stromeyer to be followed.

The tendons of the muscles which maintain the deformity should be divided with as little injury as possible to the skin and neighbouring parts.

No attempt should be made to force the foot into its natural shape immediately after the operation; but the necessary extension for that purpose should be commenced as soon as the external punctures are completely healed; this occurs about the second or third day.

The lymph which is effused between the ends of the divided tendon or tendons, with the muscles that are not divided, and the ligaments and fasciae which may impede the replacement of the foot, must be gradually extended until the foot assumes its natural shape, and the ankle can be bent to its fullest extent.

The application of the apparatus by which extension is effected must be continued for a certain period after the cure, notwithstanding that the patient has been enabled to stand firmly, and has improved in walking, in order to obviate the tendency to contraction evinced by the intermediate substance or lymph effused between the ends of the divided tendon.

Little quotes the technique of tenotomy from Stromeyer:

The operation must invariably be effected by puncture, without external incision. A very small cutting instrument should be selected—a small, moderately curved, sharp-pointed bistoury is adapted for most occasions. The limb should be extended, in order to produce the necessary projection of the tendon, when the instrument should be passed behind it, the point perforating the opposite skin; division of the tense resisting tendon being effected rather by pressure of the edge than by its slow and cautious onward movement. The skin, being elastic, yields to the pressure of the knife, the two punctures not exceeding its width. I have frequently divided the tendo Achillis in this manner without producing a second puncture; but this is of little moment, as two minute punctures heal as quickly as a single one. The division of the tendon is known by an accompanying sound, which can scarcely be mistaken. The performance of the operation with the point of the instrument is less to be relied on, partly from its being too weak, and also because the operator can be less certain of not causing injury to other structures in the event of the patient not remaining quiet throughout the operation. . . . The attempt to commence extension directly after the operation, and the endeavour immediately to restore the limb to its natural position, which will very seldom succeed, and, as the case of Sartorius proves, can only be effected by great force, is neither necessary nor advisable. The commencement of extension before cicatrisation of the wound in the integuments is unadvisable even when possible, as it may produce inflammation and suppuration not confined to the vicinity of the wound; it is unnecessary, inasmuch as the tension of the divided muscle is not restored during the gradual mechanical extension applied subsequently to the healing of the wound, but occurs after the complete reunion of the tendon and after the necessary motions of the limb during exercise have acted as a stimulus to its contractility.

Tendon Transplantation: Sir Robert Jones, 1857-1933

Robert Jones is a name that keeps recurring in British orthopaedics because he built up a school of orthopaedics, because he built up a system of organisation for the care of orthopaedic patients, and because he made many contributions over the whole field. Most of all he is remembered because he was liked, and popularity provides opportunities denied other men.

Robert's father, destined by the family to be a prosperous architect, threw up everything to write, and in consequence was poor and found it difficult to support his children. When Robert was 16, he went from his home in London to live with his uncle Hugh Owen Thomas in Liverpool, who sent him to Medical School. He had been there before with his brother on a famous occasion when he and his brothers had decided to become sailors. Robert's father had asked Thomas what he should do about this. Thomas, who had shares in some ships, put the boys on the ship with the most disagreeable captain. Robert's brother took a gun to shoot birds, but at an early stage in the voyage put a shot through the mate's hat. If the result of that did not put them off the sea, a storm shortly afterwards did so. They did not complete the voyage but landed prematurely and Robert was pleased to look forward to a medical career.

He qualified in 1878, and worked part-time with Thomas, in general practice, until the latter's death in 1891. He was appointed General Surgeon to the Royal Southern Hospital, Liverpool, in 1899, but restricted himself to orthopaedics from 1905. In the early nineties he organised and administered the Casualty Service of the Manchester Ship Canal.

In 1900 Agnes Hunt opened the Basechurch Home. It was a farmhouse and stables in which she looked after a few crippled children. When they needed surgery, she sent them to Liverpool. In 1903 her own stiff hip began to give trouble and she consulted Robert Jones. Soon afterwards she interested him in these children and from this small informal beginning there grew the Robert Jones and Agnes Hunt Orthopaedic Hospital at Oswestry, serving most of the centre of England and Wales.

When the First World War broke out Jones was aged 57—a man whose reputation was international. At first he cared for 500 orthopaedic casualties at Alder Hey, and published an excellent book on Injuries to Joints in 1916. He quickly ascended the military hierarchy and became Director General of Military Orthopaedics, and organised a scheme for disabled Service men at Shepherd's Bush.

Soon after the war ended, he put the camaraderie which had been engendered to good use, forming the British Orthopaedic Association, and set out on the third stage of his career. He had shown the path for the overall care of crippled children at Basechurch, and for disabled Service men at Shepherd's Bush; he now set himself the task of a national scheme for the detection, treatment and training of cripples. He helped found the Central Council for the Care of Cripples, and altered everyone's approach to the problem.

> "If I were made dictator, I would have an accident centre in each large city, where cases could be properly treated, and for as long as necessary. I would have beds for adults in each orthopaedic hospital and small county hospitals to act as casualty clearing stations."

His literary output was considerable, averaging about four papers a year on every aspect of orthopaedics, and it is difficult to select one particular extract for inclusion.

Robert Jones' original contributions were few. John Ridlon said that he made Thomas' teachings acceptable. But he did much more than this, he made orthopaedics a specialty.

Robert Jones' Rules for Tendon Transplantation

His rules appear in several forms and demonstrate the rapid changes in attitude that occurred in the first few years of the century. The rules he enunciated in 1908 are given first, and then a later edition of them prepared for his textbook of orthopaedics by McMurray in 1921.

1908 *Version*

In tendon transplantation one must insist on:
   1. The over-correction of deformity as a preliminary measure.

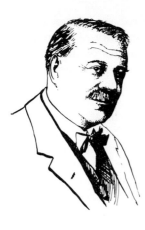

2. The removal of skin flaps to secure uninterrupted continuity of the over-correction.

Ellipses of skin were removed from the paralysed side of a joint and the incision closed to hold the over-corrected position.

3. The direct and not angular deflection of the tendon.
4. The free tunnelling in the one plane through soft tissues.
5. The firm suturing into periosteum or bony groove.
6. The careful choice, tension, and nursing of the transplanted tendon.
7. The maintenance of the hypercorrected position until voluntary power is assured to the tendon.
8. The deflection of body weight during walking from the reinforcing tendon.

In addition to these, it may sometimes be well to shorten the paralysed tendons and prevent the overaction of their opponents by tenotomy.

All my hospital transplantations are treated as out-patients, and return to their homes on the day of operation, and no difficulties of any kind arise therefrom.

1921 *Version*

Certain rules for tendon transplantation:

First: The joints upon which the transplanted tendons are called upon to act must be rendered as mobile as possible.

Second: The muscle and tendon for transplantation must be of sufficient strength to accomplish the action for which it is to be employed.

Third: The transplanted muscle and tendon must pursue a straight course between its origin and its insertion, and should not work obliquely or round an angle.

Fourth: The transplanted muscle must be attached under slight tension.

Tendon Surgery

Tendon Transplantation, A Review: J. Hilton Waterman, 1902

Probably the first man who ever grafted a tendon for any cause was Missa. The case which was reported in the Gazette Salutaire, 1770. No. 21, was as follows: The extensor of the middle finger having been severed, with resulting inability to suture it, Missa implanted the central end into the tendon of the index finger, while the peripheral end was similarly grafted upon the tendon of the ring finger. Thus, two muscles were able to exert their functions upon the wounded finger.

In a discussion upon tendon-grafting before the Paris Surgical Society in 1874, Polaillon announced that he grafted a tendon in 1873. The patient had ruptured the three middle extensor tendons of one hand. Polaillon cut down three days later and found the central ends retracted beyond the possibility of suture. He merely attached the peripheral ends to the tendons of the thumb and little finger. The patient was able to extend the finger, but adhesions formed between the cicatrix and the tendons.

In 1874 Tillaux reported a case of tendon-grafting before the Paris Surgical Society. He operated two months after the division of the tendons of the little and ring fingers, the external wound having healed. Upon cutting down the usual retraction of the central ends was found. The extensor tendon of the medius was then incised longitudinally and the peripheral ends of the two severed tendons were grafted therein, after freshening their edges. The tendons were fastened by a metallic suture. The cutaneous wound was then closed and the hand placed in a retentive apparatus. Two and a half months later the fingers could be flexed and extended. The only drawback to a perfect result was the adhesion of the operation scar to the tendons.

One year later (1875) both Duplay and Tillaux reported cases of tendon-grafting before the Paris Surgical Society. Duplay's patient was seen for the first time six weeks after the division of the extensor tendons of the thumb, which remained in the position of flexion. As suture was out of the question, the extensor carpi radialis was incised, and the peripheral end of the tendon of the extensor longus pollicis was affixed therein by a metallic suture. The result was almost perfect. If the thumb were folded into the palm it could be voluntarily extended. Tillaux, in discussion, stated that he had performed the same operation with a good result a few days before.

After reading these cases we receive the impression that probably all surgeons at the time of the publication of Velpeau's work must have been aware of the practicability of tendon-grafting. Valentine Mott, who translated and edited Velpeau's work, was necessarily aware of this surgical resource and, through him, the American surgeons of his day. In the short discussions before the Paris Surgical Society, ordinary tendon-suture was spoken of as a relatively common procedure, while grafting or suture by anastomosis, as it was called, was stated to be an exceedingly rare event. This leads me to state that the term "grafting" is of recent origin, for in the old cases which I have cited, the operation is called tendon-anastomosis, or suture by anastomosis.

It appears reasonable to suppose that tendon transplantation has been done in the past more generally than is believed to have been the case. Doubtless a study of the entire literature of tendon-suture would reveal the existence of cases similar to those just described. It seems probable that Nicoladoni or his associates may have been aware of the existence of successful cases of this sort, although this author remains absolutely silent upon this point. It is certainly not a very wide leap from grafting for the functional impotence induced by old traumatic separation of a muscle and the same operation done for paralysis of central origin.

In April, 1881, Nicoladoni showed before the Surgical Section at the annual meeting of the Society of German Naturalists and Physicians a sixteen-year-old boy whom he had recently operated upon for paralytic talipes calcaneus. As all the calf muscles were paralysed, the tendons of the two peroneal muscles were divided and the central ends were implanted into a longitudinal split in the tendo Achillis. The author was able to show the members of the Society that the contraction of the peroneal muscles produced plantar flexion of the foot, while the patient's gait was considerably improved.

During the following year Nicoladoni reported this case in great detail. As a brief review of the particulars of this case of grafting for paralysis will bring out a series of practical points, I shall enumerate its more salient features: the patient was able to execute dorsal flexion, while plantar flexion was impossible. He could not flex the great toe; the second toe moved but slightly in the attempt to flex it, while the three outside toes could be readily flexed. In the effort to flex his toes the foot was placed in dorsal flexion while the periphery of the foot was arched toward the heel, and during these movements the peronei were felt to contract. Faradic examination showed a prompt reaction on the part of the tibialis anticus, extensor hallucis, extensor communis digitorum and both peronei. No reaction in any of the calf muscles was obtained and only a very weak response from the muscles of the sole of the foot. In view of the complete absence of plantar flexion it occurred to Nicoladoni to implant the tendons of the healthy peronei into the tendo Achillis. An incision was made over the peronei tendons, which were cut through while some of the muscular origin was detached from the fibula. A second incision at right angles to the first exposed the tendo Achillis. On carrying the dissection upward the belly of the gastro-onemius was found to be completely transformed into fat. An oblique incision was made lengthwise in the tendo Achillis, so as to provide a sort of mortise for the reception of the tendons of the peronei, thereby securing a large adhesion surface. Sutures were applied and as a precautionary measure, the bellies of the peronei were sutured to the integument to prevent retraction which would tear apart the tendon-suture.

Very soon after performing this operation Nicoladoni was appointed to the chair of surgery at the University of Innsbruck, so that the case passed from his care. During the exercises of a long and active career it does not appear that this surgeon ever took up this operation a second time. While the immediate results in the first case were very promising, it is stated by Maydl that the anastomosis finally separated and all the benefits of the operation were forfeited.

The Nicoladoni operation, as it was called, was performed in four or five other cases by Von Hacker, Maydl and some of the other surgeons attached to Albert's clinic, invariably for pes calcaneus, but the ultimate results appear to have been disappointing. No attempt was made to extend the operation to other forms of paralytic deformities, and it is apparent that as early as 1886, the operation of tendon-grafting had been definitely abandoned by the German and Austrian surgeons. So little activity resulted from these operations that a few years later, when this mode of intervention was rediscovered independently by a number of surgeons, some time elapsed before Nicoladoni's brilliant efforts in this direction were duly recognised.

The first American surgeons to report cases of tendon transplantation were Milliken and Parrish of New York. Announcing (as did Nicoladoni) that they had introduced a new and original principle into surgery, Parrish explains how he was led to perform his operation. First, he remarked upon the great frequency of talipes valgus following infantile paralysis. He then calls attention to the fact that in the vast majority of these cases the tibialis anticus alone is paralysed, while the extensor longus pollicis retains its strength.

After experimenting upon the cadaver, Parrish became convinced that his principle was both correct and practicable. His first operation was performed in May, 1892. The patient was about four years old and had been paralysed for nearly three years. Of the various muscles originally involved, all had regained their functions save the tibialis anticus and posticus, paralysis of which had caused talipes valgus. The foot could be replaced in its natural position and the extensor longus pollicis was moderately strong.

This author made an incision over the tendons of the anterior tibial and extensor longus pollicis. The tendons were found and isolated, the sheaths cut away, the foot placed in inversion and extension to shorten the tendon of the tibialis anticus and pull down that of the extensor longus pollicis. The opposing tendinous surfaces were then freshened and coapted for an inch or more with catgut sutures. The foot was immobilised for a month in a plaster-of-Paris dressing. The result in this case is not clearly outlined, but the inference is that it was not brilliant.

Parrish speaks as if he had operated on other cases of the same character, although he gives no details. His procedure was a distinct advance over that of Nicoladoni in that he did not sacrifice anything; he made one muscle do the work of another without abandoning its own function. In conclusion he expresses the belief that transplantation will find its principal use in talipes valgus with a possibility of extension to the treatment of pes calcaneus. It does not appear that this American surgeon continued his brilliant work on this subject. His efforts, like those of Nicoladoni, appear to have lacked immediate results.

The next independent report of value of tendon transplantation in infantile paralysis was written by Drobnik, a Polish surgeon. While this operation was a mere episode in the practice of his predecessors —something to be taken up only to be dropped again—Drobnik continued to develop the method until he was able to report sixteen cases. While those before him—with the possible exception of Von

Hacker—had never reported a truly successful ultimate result, Drobnik obtained a number which were extremely brilliant. While his predecessors reported little or no attempt to extend the operation of transplantation to affections other than the different forms of paralytic equinovarus, Drobnik made use of the method in paralysis of the upper extremity. He states that in 1892, he became impressed with the inutility of the treatment of paralytic clubfoot in comparison with the good results obtained in the ordinary congenital variety. His first patient was a case of marked equinovarus paralyticus upon which every resource of treatment had been exhausted. She walked upon the outer edge of the dorsum of the foot. The only muscle paralysed appeared to be the extensor communis digitorum. The peronei were simply atrophic from the stretching to which they were being subjected, and gave a weak reaction. The child wore a brace which was very troublesome and the parents decided to have a tenotomy of the tendo Achillis performed. Two weeks later Drobnik operated again, divided the tendon of the extensor hallucis and implanted the central end into the tendon of the paralysed extensor communis digitorum, the position of the foot having been corrected. The result in this case was excellent, the patient being enabled finally to use skates without discomfort.

His second case was a duplicate of that operated on by Parrish and treated by the same method of grafting, save that he divided the tendon of the extensor longus pollicis outright. Drobnik's third patient had a pes calcaneus. The tendo Achillis was freshened on either side and a segment from both the flexor longus digitorum and the peronei was sutured thereto.

The fifth case is of special interest, as it is the first recorded example of grafting for infantile paralysis of the upper extremity. The only muscles which retained their functions were the two extensor carpi radiales. The extensor longus was implanted outright upon the extensor communis digitorum, while one half of the short extensor was sutured to the extensor longus pollicis. The patient regained through this operation considerable use of the fingers.

Numerous other cases reported by Drobnik are of interest but no new principles are introduced.

Another writer who advocated tendon transplantation in paralytic equinovarus was Phocas, who operated upon a single case in 1893. His patient had paralysis of the tibialis anticus and posticus with resulting pes valgus. The calf muscles were weak. He divided the tibialis anticus, sutured the peripheral end to the central stump of the extensor longus pollicis, while the central end of the tibialis anticus was sutured to the peripheral end of the extensor longus pollicis.

Still another operator was Winklemann, who operated in 1894 upon a case of peroneal paralysis, splitting the tendo Achillis into two segments, one of which he grafted upon the cut peripheral end of the peroneal tendons.

The next surgeon chronologically to take up tendon transplantation for infantile paralysis was Goldthwait of Boston, about 1894. Like his immediate predecessors, Goldthwait started with the impression that the method was original. He took the interest to look into the literature in connection with his admirable work on this subject and learned of the case of Nicoladoni and "one or two other cases abroad with a few in America." The latter probably represent the experience of Parrish. In his first case, one of pes calcaneo-valgus, he grafted the peroneus longus upon the tendo Achillis and the peroneus brevis on the flexor longus pollicis. This and three other cases reported at the time illustrate no advances in principle or technic over those of the other operators, but I shall have occasion to refer to Goldthwait's brilliant work later, in connection with the introduction of direct muscle transplantation into these operations.

Next comes the work of Franke, which marks a new epoch in tendon transplantation. This author was the first to bring about an innovation, namely, the application of this method to infantile spastic paralysis of cerebral origin. The credit for this is often mentioned as belonging to Eulenburg, but it appears that Franke preceded him by some two years. A second innovation due to this surgeon is a composite procedure for the treatment of radial paralysis in which tendon transplantation represents an important feature.

Franke's first case of cerebral paralysis occurred in a six-year-old boy who suffered at the age of one year from acute encephalitis. As a result he developed athetosis and paralysis of the right leg and arm. The foot was in the position of equinovarus. The entire muscular power of the lower extremity was weak, the peronei were paralysed and the extensors of the toes were paretic. As the tibialis anticus was strong, the peripheral portion of the tendon of the extensor longus digitorum was grafted into it. The improvement obtained was very satisfactory. The gait was more certain and the patient could walk without stumbling. While this case was unlike those previously reported in being of cerebral instead of spinal origin, it does not appear to have exhibited any element of spastic paralysis.

Franke afterward reported a case of eminently spastic paralysis as follows: The patient was a boy aged nine years who had had an equinovarus since infancy. Examination showed that the flexors, though intact, were the seat of violent contractions, while the extensors and peronei were in a state of paresis. The boy exhibited athetoid movements of the hand of the same side. In this case he first lengthened the tendo Achillis to overcome the equinus. The foot was then put in a plaster-of-Paris dressing, but when this was removed some spasm of the toes was still present. The next step was to tenotomise the flexor longus digitorum, but the contractions still persisted. This phenomenon could only be explained by the presence of an anastomosis between the tendons of the flexor longus pollicis and flexor longus digitorum, such as occasionally occurs. The flexor longus pollicis was then tenotomised and all spasms practically ceased. Transplantation of the tendo Achillis upon the peronei proved to be a useful step in the treatment of the case, but some correction became necessary, so the tendons of the peronei were cut, the foot corrected and again placed in plaster of Paris. As a result of all these successive interventions, the foot was restored to normal position and the gait was much improved. Some very slight spasm of the toes remained, but not sufficient to demand further surgical attention.

Credit for suggesting and carrying out tendon transplantation in infantile cerebral spastic paralysis must also be given to Eulenburg, the distinguished neurologist of Berlin, who appears to have been the first in his special department to foresee the great possibilities of this form of intervention in paralysis. In fact, Eulenburg goes even further in his statements than the other surgeons, for he sees no limit to the usefulness of this operation in paralysis, predicting that it will soon be employed in hemiplegia and peripheral palsies of all kinds. Eulenburg's case was an example of cerebral diplegia or so-called Little's disease. The peculiar muscular contractions made walking an impossibility. The child was four years old and the precise deformity was equinovarus of a spastic nature. The tendo Achillis was partly transplanted into the peroneal tendons, and the foot was then overcorrected after tenotomy of the remaining half of the tendo Achillis. The result in this case was surprisingly good.

I shall next proceed to discuss Franke's improved method of procedure in arm paralysis. As may be recalled, Drobnik was the first to operate for this condition, the case consisting of partial radial paralysis. Franke's case was one of total radial paralysis, a much more serious affection. While Drobnik was able to make use of two sound extensor muscles for grafting, Franke could employ but a single muscle for this purpose.

In the treatment of radial paralysis we must restore to the hand its power of extension. This could not be effected by mere transplantation of tendons. Franke's operation was performed as follows: The patient, who was eight years of age, lost almost the entire use of her arm when in the second year of her life, following a febrile attack. The arm was frail and there was marked atrophy, the picture being typical of total radial paralysis. The first step consisted in the shortening of the tendon of the extensor carpi radialis longus. The sheaths of the tendons of both the extensor and flexor carpi ulnaris were opened. As this flexor possessed some power, its tendon was divided and the central end implanted into the tendon of the extensor communis digitorum at the point where the latter becomes fan-shaped. The flexor tendon was made to occupy the groove of the extensor; in this case, therefore, a flexor muscle was made to do the work of an antagonist. The transplanted muscle was made tense and the dressing applied with the hand placed in a position of marked extension. After the wound had healed it was found that the child could extend as well as flex her fingers.

The next step consisted of an arthrodesis of the shoulder joint to prevent the rotation of the arm inward. In analysing the result it appears that the flexor carpi ulnaris extends both the fingers and the hand. The fingers can be extended beyond the horizontal position and the child can also extend the hand when it has been flexed beneath the horizontal position. With such a result Franke felt confident that radial paralysis would be no longer an incurable affection

In 1895 Krynski reported a case of grafting for traumatic separation of the flexor tendon of the middle finger. As the central end could not be reached, he implanted the peripheral portion into the tendon of the neighbouring index finger. This case is regarded as a natural outgrowth of the Nicoladoni operation, yet as we have abundantly observed, it is merely the same procedure advised under such circumstances by Velpeau and Malgaigne.

In 1897 Kirsch reported a similar case in which he buttonholed the peripheral ends of the cut extensors of the thumb into the extensor carpi radialis longus. Curiously enough this author appears to have been quite unaware of the new school of tendon transplantation, but he was conversant with some of the older cases reported before Nicoladoni's time, and it is through the clue thus furnished that I have been aided in locating those cases operated upon in past years.

There still remains for discussion an additional stage in the development of tendon transference. I refer to the direct transplantation of muscle tissue. This, as far as I know, was first done by Goldthwait in 1895. Noticing that the sartorius generally escapes paralysis in those cases of anterior poliomyelitis which involve the thigh, he conceived the idea of making this muscle do the work of the paralysed quadriceps. All previous transplantation had been done with muscles having well-formed tendons. The lower extremity of the sartorius muscle was attached to the quadriceps extensor just above the patella. He has done the operation a number of times and has secured some excellent results, the flinging gait and rotation having been obviated.

5 REDUCTIONS

Reduction of a Dislocated Shoulder: Hippocrates, 3rd Century B.C.

Of all that has been written on orthopaedics, the message of this short account is perhaps best known and least altered:

> In all dislocations, reduction is to be effected if possible immediately, while still warm, but otherwise, as quickly as it can be done; for reduction will be a much quicker and easier process for the operator, and a much less painful one to the patient, if effected before swelling comes on.
>
> Those who attempt reduction with the heel operate in a manner which is an approach to the natural. The patient must lie on the ground on his back, while the person who is to effect the reduction is seated upon the ground on the side of the dislocation; then the operator, seizing with his hand the affected arm, is to pull it, while with his heel in the armpit he pushes in the contrary direction, the right heel being placed in the right armpit, and the left heel in the left armpit. But a round ball of suitable size must be placed in the hollow of the armpit; the most convenient are very small and hard balls, formed from several pieces of leather sewn together. For without something of this kind the heel cannot reach to the head of the humerus, since, when the arm is stretched, the armpit becomes hollow, the tendons on both sides of the armpit making counter-contraction so as to oppose the reduction. But another person should be seated on the other side of the patient to hold the sound shoulder, so that the body may not be dragged along when the arm of the affected side is pulled; and then, when the ball is placed in the armpit, a supple piece of thong sufficiently broad is placed around it, and some person taking hold of its two ends is to seat himself above the patient's head to make counter extension, while at the same time he pushes with his foot against the bone at the top of the shoulder. The ball should be placed as much inside as possible, upon the ribs, and not upon the head of the humerus.

Hippocrates on Recurrent Dislocation of the Shoulder: 3rd Century B.C.

Those who are subject to frequent dislocations at the shoulder joint, are for the most part competent to effect reduction themselves; for having introduced the knuckles of the other hand into the armpit, they force the joint upwards, and bring the elbow towards the breast.

It deserves to be known how a shoulder which is subject to frequent dislocations should be treated. For many persons, owing to this accident, have been obliged to abandon gymnastic exercises, though otherwise well qualified for therein; and from the same misfortune have become inept in warlike practices and have thus perished. And this subject deserves to be noticed because I have never known any physician treat the case properly. For many physicians have burned the shoulder subject to dislocation at the top of the shoulder, at the anterior part . . . and a little behind the top of the shoulder: these burnings, if the dislocations of the arm were upwards, or forwards, or backwards would have been properly performed; but now when the dislocation is downwards, they promote rather than prevent dislocations, for they shut out the head of the humerus from the free space above.

The cautery should be applied thus: taking hold of the skin of the armpit, it is drawn into the line in which the head of the humerus is dislocated, and then the skin thus drawn aside is to be burnt to the opposite side. The burnings should be performed with irons . . . When you have burnt through, it will be sufficient in most cases to make eschars only in the lower part, but if there is a considerable piece of skin between the holes, a thin spatula may be passed through the holes and the skin is let go. Then between the two eschars you should form another eschar with a slender iron, and burn through until you come in contact with the spatula.

The following directions will enable you to determine how much skin of the armpit should be grasped; all men have glands in the armpit. The glands should not be taken hold of, nor the parts internal to the glands; for this would be attended with great danger as they are adjacent to the most important nerves. But the greater part of the substances external to the glands are to be grasped, for there is no danger from them. You should only raise the arm a little and grasp a large quantity of skin. The nerves which you ought to guard against are left within and at a distance from the operation.

When the sores have become clean and are going on to cicatrisation, then by all means the arm is bound to the side night and day; and even when the ulcers are completely healed the arm must still be bound to the side for a long time; for thus more especially will cicatrisation take place, and the wide space into which the humerus used to escape will be contracted.

Kocher's Manoeuvre: Theodor Kocher, 1841-1917

Kocher was one of the most brilliant surgeons of his day, who combined a mastery of basic principles, an enquiring mind, and superb operating technique, which was recognised by the award of the Nobel Prize for Medicine in 1909.

He was born in Berne, and studied in Berlin, London, Paris and Vienna, graduating from Berne in 1865. He became Professor of Surgery there in 1872. During the whole of his life he maintained an interest in surgical anatomy and surgical approaches; most days he would work out approaches on cadavers. This had two orthopaedic consequences: he worked out a rational technique for relaxing the muscles around the shoulder and easing a dislocated shoulder into position. One day he was in the audience watching Billroth and his firm trying to reduce a shoulder dislocation without success. Kocher asked if he could try his newly reasoned method. He succeeded, and later published his technique in 1870.

The other consequence of his study of surgical approaches was a remarkable book, which has been translated into English, describing a tremendous variety of incisions, many of which remain classical. It is well worth consulting.

One feels that Kocher only used orthopaedics to sharpen his wits for his main interest—thyroid disease, to which he contributed so much. In addition he wrote widely and deeply on many topics, and invented surgical instruments as he needed them, without thinking it anything but commonplace.

When he died Moynihan wrote an epitaph worth bearing in mind: he had a "freedom from prejudice for his own intellectual progeny".

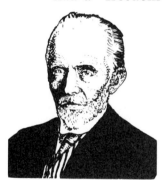

Kocher's method of reduction of a dislocated shoulder: 1870

Method:

> Bend the arm at the elbow, press it against the body, rotate outwards till a resistance is felt, lift the externally rotated upper arm in the sagittal plane as far as possible forwards, and finally turn inwards slowly.

This is taken from a long closely reasoned article confusingly illustrated by six engravings some of which are printed upside down.

Kocher worked out his technique on cadavers. He aimed at bringing the greater tuberosity of the humerus into contact with the glenoid rim to act as a fulcrum. This was achieved by flexing the externally rotated shoulder, which also relaxed the upper anterior part of the capsule that would otherwise form a tense cord. When the arm is internally rotated the head pivots on the fulcrum and slips into the glenoid.

Kocher claimed these advantages of the method—it was painless because movements were not forced, and did not require either anaesthesia or assistants. It was only suitable for subcoracoid dislocations with three provisos—that capsular damage was not so extensive that the bone surfaces were not held apposed, that neither the glenoid rim nor the greater tuberosity were fractured which would also prevent them pivoting one on the other.

Reduction of a Fracture of the Neck of the Femur: Guy Whitman Leadbetter, 1893-1945

Leadbetter was born in Bangor, Maine, and studied at Bowdoin College, where he established a record for throwing the hammer, before graduating from Johns Hopkins in 1920. While a student he decided to become an orthopaedic surgeon and after three years training set up in private practice in Washington, D.C. He quickly established his reputation, one of his principal interests being fractures of the neck of the femur. Later he became Professor of Surgery at George Washington Medical School.

He was a man of stern appearance and serious mind, a man with a wide range of interests, efficient and modest. He was a pianist, a linguist, amateur archaeologist and also gave lectures on the background of the Nation's Parks.

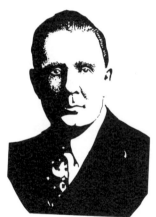

The Leadbetter Manoeuvre: 1933

Anatomical reposition of the fragments is the only position which insures good union and good function.

The manipulation suggested here is simple, anatomically sound, non-shocking, and offers opportunity for 100% reduction. The patient is first anaesthetised, usually with ethylene gas, on the fracture table. The uninjured leg is harnessed to the foot stirrup. The injured leg is then flexed at the hip at ninety degrees, with the lower leg at ninety degrees to the thigh. Direct manual traction in the axis of the flexed thigh is then made, together with slight adduction of the femoral shaft. In this position the thigh is internally rotated approximately forty-five degrees. The leg is slowly circumducted into abduction, the internally rotated position being maintained. The amount of abduction varies with the individual and can be measured accurately, representing the difference in degrees of the angle made by the fractured neck with the shaft and the angle between the neck and the shaft on the normal side, as evidenced by the roentgengram.

The test which in our experience has indicated that the fracture has been completely reduced is as follows. After the leg has been brought down in the measured degree of abduction and internal rotation, the heel of the injured leg is allowed to rest on the outstretched palm. If the reduction is complete, the leg will not evert itself. Should there be no interlocking of the fragments, however, the leg will slowly rotate externally. This has been found to be an invariable test.

Leadbetter read this paper in 1932 in the days before these fractures were nailed. After reduction patients were encased in plaster from nipple to toe. It is interesting to notice his results. Of 31 intracapsular fractures, 4 died (one pulmonary embolus, one diabetic coma, one cellulitis of neck, and one renal infection), twenty-two united, seven went to nonunion and two underwent absorption. Most people today would be pleased if 70 per cent. of their intracapsular fractures united.

CODA

Is it useful to look back on the past? Even a cursory study of history saves one discovering ideas and data afresh for oneself. So much of medical new thinking is an inadvertent repetition of old thinking. This may be good for the soul but is rather a waste of time if it goes beyond arm-chair philosophising. Perhaps this recollection of old writing may show that there is much worth consulting. Every generation must have its fashion—but everything that is old is not old-fashioned. Every trend setter of today will at the very best be remembered by an operation that has been outdated, a physical sign that has been improved upon or a disease that he ill understood. Even his real message will probably be misrepresented.

If we go a few years into the past, we find the state of affairs that we are reacting against today. It can be understood. Go a few years further and all is unfamiliar. The ideas are original again.

Appendix: How to find biographies, portraits, and original papers

1. *Biographies*

The dates, occupation, and nationality of most of the memorable doctors can be found in the *Encyclopaedia of Medical Sources* by E. R. Kelly and published by Williams and Wilkins, Baltimore, 1948.

Short biographical notes may be found in standard works on Medical History such as Garrison, Guthrie, Major or Nettler.

Biographical information may be had from obituaries. When the date of death has been learnt from Kelly the reference to an obituary may be found in a medical index. The *Surgeon General's Catalogue* is best up to 1932 after which the *Index Medicus* is better.

Commemorative biographies are published in the Journals from time to time and these may be found in the *Index Medicus*.

Fellows of the College of Surgeons of England are included in a series of volumes published by the College under the title of *Lives of the Fellows*. This carries many references to other biographies and portraits.

At the Wellcome Historical Medical Library there is a bibliographical card index with very up-to-date information.

2. *Portraits*

Some obituaries include portraits: the *Surgeon General's Catalogue* indicates this. Standard medical histories include many portraits. The Wellcome Historical Medical Library and the Royal Society of Medicine have photographic and print collections of portraits; copies may be requested.

3. *Original Papers*

There is a recognised corpus of original papers. The reference to these may be found in the following:-

    a) *Encyclopaedia of Medical Sources* by E. R. Kelly, Baltimore, Williams & Wilkins, 1948.

    b) *A Medical Bibliography* by L. T. Morton, London, Grafton 1954.

    c) *Source Book of Orthopaedics* by E. M. Bick, Baltimore, Williams & Wilkins, 1948.

    d) *Menders of the Maimed* by Arthur Keith, London, OUP, 1919.

A great deal of material has not been catalogued and is easily but slowly unearthed in a long established library.

When the reference has been found, the next task is to locate the journal. This may be learned from the *World List of Scientific Periodicals*; most libraries will send inexpensive photocopies on application.

The history of orthopaedics has been described very well in two books both of which are out of print.
BICK, E. M. (1948). *Source book of Orthopaedics.* Baltimore: Williams & Wilkins.
KEITH, A. (1919). *Menders of the Maimed.* London: Oxford University Press.

Part 2. Classic Descriptions of Disease

INFECTIONS

Spinal Tuberculosis
> HIPPOCRATES (1849). *Genuine Works of Hippocrates.* Translated by F. Adams. London:
> New Sydenham Society.

Tuberculous Paraplegia
> POTT, P. (1808). Remarks on that kind of palsy of the lower limbs. *Chirurgical Works of Pott.*
> London: Wood & Innes. (Also published as Pamphlet in 1779.)

Brodie's Abscess
> BRODIE, Sir B. (1832). *Med. Chir. Trans.* **17**, 239.

Tom Smith's Arthritis of Infancy
> SMITH, Sir T. (1874). *St Bart's Hosp. Rep.* **10**, 189-204.

BONE DISEASE

Paget's Disease
> PAGET, Sir J. (1877). *Med. Chir. Trans.* **60**, 37-64.
> PAGET, Sir J. (1882). *Med. Chir. Trans.* **65**, 225.

Dyschondroplasia
> OLLIER, L. (1900). Lyon méd. **93**, 23-5. (Translated by Helen Rang.)

Melorheostosis
> LÉRI, A. & JOANNY (1922). *Bull. Soc. Méd. Hôp. Paris.* **46**, 1141-5. (Translated by Helen Rang.)
> LÉRI, A. & LIÈVRE, J. A. (1928). *Pr. méd.* **36**, 801.
> LÉRI, A., LOISELEUR & LIÈVRE (1930). *Bull. Soc. Méd. Hôp. Paris.* **54**, 1210-7.

Subungual Exostosis
> DUPUYTREN, Baron G. (1847). *Injuries and diseases of bones.* Translated by F. Le Gros Clark,
> p. 410. London: New Sydenham Society.

JOINT DISEASE

Internal Derangement of the Knee
> HEY, W. (1803). *Practical Observations in Surgery,* Chap. 8. London: Capell.

Baker's Cyst
> BAKER, W. MORRANT (1877). *St Bart's Hosp. Rep.* **13**, 245-261.
> BAKER, W. MORRANT (1885). *St Bart's Hosp. Rep.* **21**, 177-190.

Hoffa's Disease
> HOFFA, A. (1904). *J. Amer. med. Ass.* **43**, 795-6.

Madelung's Deformity
> MADELUNG, O. (1878). *Verh. dtsch. Ges. Chir.* **7**, pt. 2, 259-275. (Translated by D. Pevsner.)

Still's Disease
> STILL, Sir G. (1897). *Med. Chir. Trans.* **80**, 47-59.

Charcot's Joints
> CHARCOT, J.-M. (1881). *Lectures on the diseases of the nervous system.* Translated by G. Sigerson.
> vol. **2**, p. 49-61. London: New Sydenham Society.

Neuromuscular Disease

Little's Disease

LITTLE, W. J. (1862). *Trans. Obstet. Soc. Lond.* **3,** 293.

Brachial Plexus Injuries

DUCHENNE, G. B. A. (1883). *Selection of the Clinical Works of Duchenne.* Translated by G. V. Poore. London: New Sydenham Society.

ERB, W. H. (1877). *Verh. naturh.-med. Ver. Heidelb.* N.F. Bd **1,** 130-136. (Translated by Dr. Hirsch.)

KLUMPKE, A. DÉJERINE- (1885). *Rev. Médecine.* **5,** 591-616, 739-790. (Translated by Helen Rang.)

Neurofibromatosis

SMITH, R. W. (1849). *A Treatise on the Pathology, Diagnosis & Treatment of Neuroma.* Dublin: Hodges & Smith.

Sciatica

FRIBERG, S. (1941). *Acta chir. scand.* **85,** Supplement 64.

MIXTER, W. J. & BARR, J. S. (1934). *New Engl. J. Med.* **211,** 210-214.

WALKER, A. E. (1951). *A History of Neurological Surgery.* London: Baillière.

COTUGNO, D. (1775). *A Treatise on the Nervous Sciatica.* London: Wilkie.

MIDDLETON, G. S. & TEACHER, J. H. (1911). *Glasg. med. J.* **76,** 1.

GOLDTHWAIT, J. E. (1911). *Boston med. surg. J.* **164,** 365-372.

Morton's Metatarsalgia

MORTON, T. G. (1876). *Amer. J. med. Sci.* **71,** 37-45.

DURLACHER, L. (1845). *A treatise on Corns, Bunions, and diseases of the nails, and the general management of the feet.* London: Simpkin, Marshall.

Carpal Tunnel Syndrome

MARIE, P. & FOIX, C. (1913). *Rev. neurol.* **26,** 647.

WOLTMAN, H. W. (1941). *Arch. Neurol. Psychiat.* **45,** 680.

SEDDON, H. J. in ZACHARY, R. B. (1945). *Surg. Gynec. Obstet.* **81,** 213.

BRAIN, W. RUSSELL, WRIGHT, A., DICKSON & WILKINSON, M. (1947). *Lancet,* **1,** 277-282.

PAGET, Sir J. (1853). *Lectures on Surgical Pathology,* vol. 1, p. 43. London: Longmans.

ORMEROD, J. A. (1883). *St Bart's Hosp. Rep.* **19,** 17-26.

Myositis Ossificans Progressiva

FREKE, J. (1740). *Phil. Trans.* **41,** 369-370.

Osteochondritis Juvenalis

(General)

KING, E. S. J. (1935). *Localised rarefying conditions of bone as exemplified by Legg-Perthes' disease, Osgood-Schlatter's disease, etc.* London: Arnold.

Scheuermann's Disease

SCHEUERMANN, H. W. (1921). *Z. orthopad. Chir.* **51,** 305-317. (Translated by Dr. Hirsch.)

STAFFORD, R. A. (1832). *The injuries, the diseases, and distortions of the spine.* London: Longmans.

Coxa Plana

LEGG, A. T. (1910). *Boston med. surg. J.* **162,** 202-4.

LEGG, A. T. (1916). *Surg. Gynec. Obstet.* **22,** 307-323.

PERTHES, G. (1920). *Zbl. Chir.* **47,** 123-5.

LEGG, A. T. (1918). *Amer. J. orth. Surg.* **16,** 448-52.

LEGG, A. T. (1927). *J. Bone Jt Surg.* **9,** 26-34.

Apophysitis of the Tibial Tubercle

PAGET, Sir J. (1891). *Studies of old case books,* pp. 6-7. London: Longmans.

OSGOOD, R. B. (1903). *Boston med. Surg. J.* **148,** 114-7.

Trauma

Shock

HALL, M. (1825). *Medical Essays,* pp. 37-40. London.

HALL, M. (1830). *Researches principally relative to the morbid & curative effects of loss of blood.* p. 108. London: Seeley & Burnside.

Rupture of Tendo Achillis

PARÉ, A. (1665). *The workes of that famous chirurgion Ambrose Parey.* Translated by T. Johnson, p. 284. London.

Pulled Elbow

THOMAS, H. O. (1883). *The principles of treatment of diseased joints.* p. 77. London: Lewis.

Ischaemic Contracture

VOLKMANN, R. von (1881). *Zbl. Chir.* **8,** 801-3. (Translated by J. D. Wicht.)

FRACTURES

COLLES, A. (1814). *Edinb. med. Surg. J.* **10**, 182-6.

SMITH, R. W. (1847). *A treatise on fractures in the vicinity of joints, and on certain forms of accidental and congenital dislocations*, p. 162. Dublin: Hodges & Smith.

BENNETT, E. H. (1882). *Dublin J. med. Sci.* **73**, 72-5.

MONTEGGIA, G. B. (1814). *Instituzioni Chirurgiche*, vol. 5, p. 130, para. 260. Milan: Maspero. (Translated Helen Rang.)

GALEAZZI, R. (1934). *Arch. orthop. Unfallchir.* **35**, 557-562. (Translated by D. Pevsner.)

POTT, P. (1808). Remarks on Fractures and Dislocations. *Chirurgical Works of Pott*, pp. 325-9. London: Wood & Innes.

DUPUYTREN, Baron G. (1847). *Injuries and diseases of bones*, pp. 282-3. Translated by F. Le Gros Clark. London: New Sydenham Society.

FREIBERG, A. H. (1914). *Surg. Gynec. Obstet.* **19**, 191-3.

MISCELLANEOUS

Gout

HIPPOCRATES (1849). *Genuine Works of Hippocrates.* Translated by F. Adams. London: New Sydenham Society.

SYDENHAM, T. (1850). *The Works of Thomas Sydenham.* Translated by R. G. Latham. London: New Sydenham Society.

Dupuytren's Contracture

CLINE, H. (Quoted by WINDSOR, J.). (1834). *Lancet*, **2**, 501.

COOPER, Sir A. (1822). *A treatise on dislocations and fractures of the joints*, p. 524. London: Longmans.

DUPUYTREN, Baron G. (1834). *Lancet*, **2**, 222-5.

de Quervain's Stenosing Tenovaginitis

DE QUERVAIN, F. (1895). *Korresp.-Bl. schweiz. Arz.* **25**, 389-94. (Translated by D. Pevsner.)

Vertebra Plana

CALVÉ, J. (1925). *J. Bone Jt Surg.* **7**, 41-6.

Ganglion

PAUL OF AEGINA (1846). *Paulus Aegineta.* Translated by F. Adams, **2**, 315. London: New Sydenham Society.

Ankylosing Spondylitis

COPEMAN, W. S. C. (1964). *A Short History of Gout & the Rheumatic Diseases.* Berkeley: University of California Press.

CONNOR, B. (1695). *Phil. Trans.* **19**, 21-27.

DELPECH, J. M. (1828). *De l'orthomorphie*, vol. 2. Paris: Gabon.

STRUMPELL, A. (1884). *Lehrbach der speziellen Pathologie und Therapie der Innern Krankheiten.* Leipzig: Vogel. (Translated by M. Rang.)

MARIE, P. (1898). *Rev. Médecine.* **18**, 285-315. (Translated by Helen Rang.)

Part Three: Pathology

Congenital Dislocation of the Hip

DUPUYTREN, G. (1847). *Injuries and diseases of Bones*, pp. 174-5 & 178-80. Translated by F. Le Gros Clark. London: New Sydenham Society.

Callus Formation

DUPUYTREN, G. (1847). *Ibid.*, pp. 40-44.

Part Four: Physical Signs

HEBERDEN, W. (1802). *Commentaries on the History and Cure of Diseases*, pp. 148-9. London: Payne.

THOMAS, H. O. (1876). *Hip, Knee and Ankle*, 2nd ed. pp. 17-19. Liverpool: Dobbs.

TRENDELENBURG, F. (1895). *Dtsch. med. Wschr.* **21**, 21-4. (R. S. M. Translation.)

ORTOLANI, M. (1937). *Paediatria*, **45**, 129-136.

ORTOLANI, M. (1948). *La Lussazione congenita dell' anca.* Bologna: Capelli. (R.N.O.H. Translation.)

GAUVAIN, Sir H. (1918). *Lancet*, **2**, 666.

MCMURRAY, T. P. (1928). *Robert Jones Birthday Volume*, p. 305. London: Oxford University Press.

FROMENT, J. (1915). *Pr. méd.* **23**, 409. (Translated by Helen Rang.)

TINEL, J. (1917). *Nerve wounds*, p. 34. Translated by F. Rothwell. Revised by C. Joll. London: Baillière.

The Lasègue Sign
LASÈGUE, C. E. (1864). *Arch. gén. méd.* **2**, 558-580.
FORST, J.-J. (1881). *Contribution à l'étude clinique de la sciatique.* Thèse pour le Doctorat en Médecine, Paris. No. 33. (Translated by Helen Rang.)
LAZAREVIC, L. K. (1880). *Srpski Arh.* **7**, 23.
LAZAREVIC, L. K. (1884). *Allg. wien. med. Ztg.* **29**, 425.
DE BEURMANN, L. (1884). *Arch. Physiol. norm. path.* **16**, 375.
DIMITRIJEVIC, D. T. (1952). *Neurology, Minneap.* **2**, 453-4.
WARTENBURG, R. (1956). *Neurology, Minneap.* **6**, 853-8.

Part Five: Treatment

Splints and Apparatus
PARÉ, A. (1665). *The workes of that famous chirurgion Ambrose Parey*, p. 285. Translated by T. Johnson. London.
POTT, P. (1808). *Chirurgical Works of Pott*, p. 313. London: Wood & Innes.
Plaster of Paris Bandages
RHAZES (Quoted by BACON). See below.
ETON, W. (1798). *Survey of the Turkish Empire*, p. 218. London.
BALLINGALL, Sir G. (1852). *Outlines of Military Surgery*, 4th ed., p. 358. Edinburgh: Black.
MATHYSEN, A. (1854). *Du Bandage plâtre et de son application dans le traitment des fractures.* Liège: Grandmont-Donders. (Translated by Helen Rang.)
General History of Plaster of Paris
MUNRO, J. K. (1935). *Brit. J. Surg.* **23**, 257-266.
BACON, L. W. (1923). *Bull. Soc. med. Hist.* **3**, 122.
Thomas Splint
THOMAS, H. O. (1876). *Hip, Knee and Ankle*, 2nd ed., p. 98. Liverpool: Dobbs.
JONES, R. (1925). *Brit. med. J.* **1**, 909-913.

TRACTION

JAMES, J. H. (Quoted by A. ROCYN JONES). *J. Bone Jt Surg.* 1953, **35B**, 661-666.
KIRSCHNER, M. (1909). *Beitr. klin. Chir.* **44**, 266-279.
BUCK, G. (1860). *N.Y. Acad. Med.* **1**, 181-2.
RUSSELL, R. HAMILTON (1924). *Brit. J. Surg.* **11**, 491-502.
Esmarch's Bandage
ESMARCH, J. F. A. Von (1876). *German Clinical Lectures*, selected by Volkman. London: New Sydenham Society.

OPERATIONS ON BONE

Corrective Osteotomy
BARTON, J. R. (1837). *Amer. J. med. Sci.* **21**, 332-40.
MAYER (Quoted by BONNEY, F. A. B.). (1853). *Lancet*, **1**, 557-8.
MACEWEN, W. (1878). *Lancet*, **1**, 449-50.
Bone Grafting
JANEWAY, H. H. (1910). *Ann. Surg.* **11**, 217-228.
PHEMISTER, D. B. (1931). *Surg. Gynec. Obstet.* **52**, 376-381.
GHORMLEY, R. K. (1933). *J. Amer. med. Ass.* **101**, 1733.
MOWLEM, R. (1944). *Lancet*, **2**, 746.
MACEWEN, W. (1881). *Proc. Roy. Soc.* **32**, 232.
MACEWEN, W. (1909). *Ann. Surg.* **1**, 959.
Internal Fixation
LANE, Sir A. (1894). *Trans. clin. Soc. Lond.* **27**, 167-175.

OPERATIONS ON JOINTS

Arthroplasty
WHITE, C. (1847). In *A System of Surgery* by M. J. Chelius. Translated and accompanied by additional notes by J. F. South, vol. 2, p. 979. London: Henry Renshaw.
WHITE, A. *Ibid.*
BARTON, J. R. (1827). *N. Amer. med. surg. J.* **3**, 279-92 & 400.
SYME, J. (1831). *Treatise on the excision of diseased joints.* Edinburgh: Black.
HODGES (1861). *The Excision of Joints.* Boston, Mass.
DAVIES-COLLEY, J. N. (1887). *Trans. clin. Soc. Lond.* **20**, 165-171.
KELLER, W. (1904). *N.Y. med. J.* **80**, 741-2.
KELLER, W. (1912). *N.Y. med. J.* **95**, 696-8.

Arthrodesis

 PARK, H. (1783). *An Account of a new method of treating diseases of the joints of the knee and elbow, in a letter to Mr. Percivall Pott*, pp. 4 & 20. London: Johnson. (The title page reads 1733 but this is a misprint.)

 ALBERT, E. (1882). *Wien. med. Pr.* **23**, 725-8. (Translated by D. Pevsner.)

OPERATIONS ON TENDONS

Tenotomy

 LITTLE, W. J. (1839). *A Treatise on the nature of Club-foot, and analagous distortions; including their treatment both with and without surgical operation.* London: Longmans.

Tendon Transplantation

 JONES, Sir R. (1908). *Brit. med. J.* **1**, 728-732.

 McMURRAY, T. P. (1921). *Orthopaedic Surgery of Injuries.* Ed. JONES, R. London: Oxford University Press.

 WATERMAN, J. H. (1902). *Med. News*, pp. 54-61.

REDUCTIONS

Shoulder

 HIPPOCRATES (1849). *Genuine Works of Hippocrates.* Translated by F. Adams. London: New Sydenham Society.

Recurrent Dislocation

 HIPPOCRATES. *Ibid.*

Kocher's Manoeuvre

 KOCHER, T. (1870). *Berl. klin. Wschr.* **7**, 101-105. (Translation by Dr. Hirsch.)

Neck of Femur

 LEADBETTER, G. W. (1933). *J. Bone Jt Surg.* **15**, 931-40.

INDEX OF BIOGRAPHIES

ALBERT
    (1900). *J. Amer. med. Ass.* **35,** 896.

BAKER
    (1896). *St Bart's Hosp. Rep.* **32,** xxxix-xlix.

BARTON
    (1955). *Clin. Orth.,* Philadelphia **6,** 3-8.

BENNETT
    (1907). *Brit. med. J.* **1,** 1575-8.
    MCNEALY, R. W. & LICHTENSTEIN, M. E. (1933). *Surg. Gynec. Obstet.* **56,** 197.

BRODIE
    HOLMES, T. (1898). *Sir Benjamin Collins Brodie.* London: Fisher, Unwin.

BUCK
    CONWAY, H. & STARK, R. B. (1953). *Plastic Surgery at the New York Hospital, with biblio-graphical notes on Gurdon Buck.* New York: Hoeber.

CALVÉ
    (1954). *J. Bone Jt Surg.* **36B,** 502-3.

CHARCOT
    GUILLAN, G. (1959). *J.-M. Charcot.* Translated by Pearce Bailey. London.

COLLES
    JONES, A. R. (1950). *J. Bone Jt Surg.* **32B,** 126-130.

COTUGNO (or COTUNNIUS)
    (1823-4). *Lancet,* 3rd Ed. **2,** 476-7.
    LEVINSON, A. (1936). *Ann. med. Hist.* **8,** 1-9.

DAVIES-COLLEY
    STEELE (1898). *Trans. Amer. orth. Ass.* **11,** 17.
    (1900). *Lancet,* **1,** 1474.
    (1901). *Med. Chir. Trans.* **84,** cvi-cix.

DUPUYTREN
    MONDOR, H. (1946). *Dupuytren,* 8th ed. Paris: Gallimard.

ERB
    TORKILDSEN, A. & ERIKSEN, T. (1935). *Arch. Neurol. Psychiat.* **33,** 842-6.

ESMARCH
    (1961). *Amer. J. Surg.* **102,** 460.
    (1963). *J. Amer. med. Ass.* **185,** 132-4.

FREIBERG
    (1940). *J. Bone Jt Surg.* **22,** 1104-5.

FROMENT
    (1946). *J. Méd. Lyon.* **26,** 745-751.

FREKE
    MOORE, N. (1918). *History of St Bartholomew's Hospital,* vol. 2, p. 633. London: Pearson.

GALEAZZI
    (1953). *J. Bone Jt Surg.* **35B,** 679-680.

GAUVAIN
    (1945). *J. Bone Jt Surg.* **27,** 342.
    (1945). *Lancet,* **1,** 162-3.

GOLDTHWAIT
    (1961). *J. Bone Jt Surg.* **43A,** 463-4.

HALL
    (HALL, C.), (1861). *Marshall Hall* by his Widow. London: Bentley.

HEBERDEN
    HEBERDEN, W. (the Younger). (1802). In *Commentaries on the History & Cure of Diseases*. London: Payne.

HEY
    PEARSON, J. (1822). *The Life of William Hey*. London: Hurst, Robinson.

HOFFA
    (1908). *Amer. J. Orthop. Philadelphia*. **6,** 7.

JONES
    WATSON, F. (1934). *Life of Sir Robert Jones*. London: Hodder & Stoughton.
    (1957). *J. Bone Jt Surg.* **39B,** 179-217.

KELLER
    (1959). *New York Times*, July 12, p. 72.
    METZ, C. (1964). Personal Communication.

KLUMPKE
    SPILLER, S. E. (1928). *Arch. Neurol. Psychiat.* **20,** 193.

KOCHER
    (1917). *Lancet*, **2,** 167.
    (1917). *Brit. med. J.* **2,** 168-9.

LANE
    TANNER, W. E. (1946). *Arbuthnot Lane, his life and work*. London: Baillière.

LEADBETTER
    (1946). *J. Bone Jt Surg.* **28,** 186-7.

LEGG
    (1939). *J. Bone Jt Surg.* **21,** 1054.
    (1939). *N. Engl. J. Med.* **221,** 436.

LERI
    (1930). *Pr. Méd.* **38,** 1339-40.

LITTLE
    (1894). *Lancet*, **2,** 168-9.

MACEWEN
    BOWMAN, A. K. (1942). *Sir William Macewen*. London: Hodge.
    JONES, A. R. (1952). *J. Bone Jt Surg.* **34B,** 123-8.

MADELUNG
    (1926). *Arch. klin. Chir.* **143,** i-vi.

McMURRAY
    (1949). *J. Bone Jt Surg.* **31B,** 618-9.

MARIE
    COHEN, H. (1953). *Proc. R. Soc. Med.* **46,** 1047-54.

MATHYSEN
    VAN ASSEN, J. & MAYERDING, H. W. (1948). *J. Bone Jt Surg.* **30A,** 1018-9.

MIDDLETON
    GOODALL, A. L. (1963). Quoted by E. M. BICK in *Clin. Orth. Philadelphia*, **26,** 4-5.

MONTEGGIA
    PELTIER, L. F. (1957). *Surgery*, **42,** 585-91.

MORTON
    (1903). *Med. Rec. (N.Y.).* **63,** 864.
    SHARPE, W. D. (1962). *Trans. Stud. Coll. Phycns Philad.* 4th ser. **29,** 137-152.

OLLIER
    (1901). *Brit. med. J.* **1,** 184.

ORMEROD
    (1926). *St Bart's Hosp. Rep.* **59,** 1-5.

ORTOLANI
    BADER, L. (1962). *Genesi ed evoluzione dell' orthopedia in Italia*, p. 420. Padova: Liviana.

OSGOOD
    (1957). *J. Bone Jt Surg.* **39A,** 726.
    OSGOOD, R. B. (1922). *Arch. Surg.* **4,** 420-33.

PAGET
    PAGET, S. (1901). *Memoirs & Letters of Sir James Paget*. London: Longmans.

PARÉ
    PACKARD, F. P. (1926). *Life and Times of Ambroise Paré*, 2nd ed. New York: Hoeber.

PARK
    POWER, Sir D'A. (1936). *Brit. J. Surg.* **24,** 267.
    OLDHAM, J. B. (1954). *Proc. R. Soc. Med.* **47,** 1056-8.

POTT
    EARLE, Sir JAMES (1808). *(Life of Pott in) Chirurgical Works of Pott.* London: Wood & Innes.
    LLOYD, G. M. (1933). *St Bart's Hosp. Rep.* **66,** 291-336

SMITH, R. W.
    PELTIER, L. F. (1959). *Surgery,* **45,** 1035-42.

SMITH, T.
    (1909). *Lancet,* **2,** 1108-11.

STILL
    (1914). *Lancet,* **2,** 56-7.

SYDENHAM
    PAYNE, J. F. (1900). *Thomas Sydenham.* London: Unwin.

SYME
    PATERSON, R. (1874). *Memorials of the Life of James Syme.* Edinburgh: Edmonston & Douglas.

TEACHER
    GOODALL, A. L. (1963). Quoted by E. M. BICK. *Clin. Orth.* Philadelphia. **26,** 4-5.

THOMAS
    LE VAY, D. (1956). *The Life of Hugh Owen Thomas.* Edinburgh: Livingstone.

TINEL
    (1952). *Bull. Soc. méd. Hôp. Paris.* **68,** 389-91.

VOLKMANN
    ROSS, J. P. (1930). *St Bart's Hosp. J.* **38,** 47.

INDEX